MYELODYSPLASTIC SYNDROMES:

APPROACH TO DIAGNOSIS AND TREATMENT

MYELODYSPLASTIC SYNDROMES

APPROACH TO DIAGNOSIS AND TREATMENT

Harold R. Schumacher, M.D.
Director, Clinical Hematology Laboratory
Hematopathology Fellowship Program
and
Professor of Pathology
University of Cincinnati Medical Center
Cincinnati, Ohio

Sucha Nand
Associate Professor of Medicine
Section of Hematology-Oncology
Loyola University of Chicago
Stritch School of Medicine
Maywood, Illinois

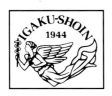

IGAKU-SHOIN   NEW YORK • TOKYO

Published and distributed by

IGAKU-SHOIN Medical Publishers, Inc.
One Madison Avenue, New York, New York 10010

IGAKU-SHOIN Ltd.,
5-24-3 Hongo, Bunkyo-ku, Tokyo 113-91.

Library of Congress Cataloging-in-Publication Data

Schumacher, Harold R. (Harold Robert)
    Myelodysplastic syndromes : approach to diagnosis and treatment /
  Harold R. Schumacher, Sucha Nand.
      p.   cm.
    Includes bibliographical references and index.
    1. Myelodysplastic syndromes.   I. Nand, Sucha.   II. Title.
    [DNLM: 1. Myelodysplastic Syndromes.   2. Bone Marrow-
  -physiopathology.   WH 380 S3915m   1995]
  RC645.73.S38   1995
  616.4'1—dc20
  DNLM/DLC
  For Library of Congress   94-13053
                                                                  CIP

ISBN: 0-89640-266-5   (New York)
ISBN: 4-260-14266-6   (Tokyo)

Printed and bound in the Hong Kong
10 9 8 7 6 5 4 3 2 1

Dedicated to
Phil and R.M. Dass

PREFACE

The primary objective of this book, like that of its sister volumes Acute and Chronic Leukemia: Approach to Diagnosis, is to provide basic, current information on the myelodysplastic syndromes (MDSs) that will allow those interested in these disorders to perfect their diagnostic and therapeutic skills in this rapidly growing area of hematology. Like the previous books, this book contains case studies that provide practical information that the diagnostician can utilize to diagnose these disorders more skillfully. Again, we have attempted to make the book succinct and totally readable, but have retained the requisite knowledge and approach to establish even the most difficult diagnosis. Also, a multifaceted, unified approach has been employed to include all pertinent information necessary to arrive at a correct diagnosis. New to this volume is a section on prognosis and treatment authored by Dr. Nand. This adds an important dimension to a complex hematopoietic disease that contains numerous conundrums related to cell biology.

Chapter 1, on the diagnostic approach, reveals some of the historical findings that led to the concept of the MDSs. In addition, it includes the contrasting features of the MDSs versus the myeloproliferative disorders (MPDs).

Chapter 2, on morphology, classification, and scoring, has great importance since one must be able to identify blast cells, dyserythropoiesis, dysgranulopoiesis, and dysmegakaryocytopoiesis to establish a diagnosis, classify the disease process, and evaluate various predictable factors.

Chapter 3, on differential diagnosis and secondary MDSs, discusses those diseases that may create the greatest difficulty in establishing the correct diagnosis, prognosis, and treatment in this group of disorders.

Chapter 4, on cytochemistry and immunohistochemistry, discusses the intermediate role of importance between the acute and chronic leukemias. How the enzyme terminal deoxynucleotidyl transferase (Tdt) functions in some cases of MDS is not known and needs further study.

Chapter 5, on transmission electron microscopy, shows the role of this imaging modality in acute and chronic leukemia.

Although immunophenotypic studies do not usually play an important major role in the diagnosis of MDS, immunological abnormalities impact heavily on these disorders. MDS patients with impaired immunity have increased susceptibility to infection, disorders in autoimmunity, and malignant neoplasms. Immunologically, they demonstrate abnormalities in immunoglobulin, B cells, T cells, NK cells, and monocytes. These topics are discussed in Chapter 6.

Cytogenetics, discussed in Chapter 7, assumes great importance since one classifies MDSs as primary (or de novo) or secondary; this is related to either an iatrogenic or an identifiable environmental toxin. The former manifest karyotypic anomalies in 40–50% of cases at diagnosis, the latter in more than 80%. Patients with secondary MDSs have a very short survival. These diseases are always associated with a trilineage myelodysplasia and fibrosis within the bone marrow biopsy.

Chapter 8, on the molecular genetic aspects of MDS, is most important since it provides insight into the cellular mechanisms operating in these disorders. MDSs originate from a pluripotent stem cell that was previously suggested by G6PD and cytogenetic investigations and established unequivocally by X-chromosome inactivation analysis. *RAS* oncogenes, mutations and deletions of the *FMS* gene, and defects in tumor-suppressor gene p53 may all be important contributors to the development of MDS. Recently, the interferon regulatory factor 1 (*IRF*-1) gene, the deleted in colorectal carcinoma gene (*DCC*), and the neurofibromatous-1 (*NF*-1) gene have been shown to play a role in the MDSs. The molecular genetic aspects of investigation are in their infancy, changing and evolving daily, and are already beginning to impact on our diagnostic and therapeutic armamentarium.

Chapter 9, on clinical features, prognosis, and treatment, emphasizes the difficulty of predicting survival and choosing appropriate therapy. This is due to the marked heterogeneity of these diseases, variable evolution patterns, imprecise knowledge of the genetic events that underlie fulminating transitions, and lack of understanding of the host factors that modulate the behavior of the individual patient.

The second portion of the book provides practical information in the case presentation format with accompanying color microphotographs. The case format provides case presentations, screening laboratory results, hospital course, questions, confirmatory laboratory results, diagnostic and therapeutic discussions, summary, answers to questions, and a current bibliography. The cases encompass simple, moderately difficult, and extremely difficult examples. The design has been created to present a logical, organized, analytical approach to the diagnosis of the MDSs.

The authors hope that this minitext will enable the reader to learn the basic and evolving complexities of diagnosis and treatment of the MDSs. This monograph is directed to the large audience of physicians who must deal with the MDSs and leukemias on a frequent basis. It is also designed to guide trainees in pathology and hematology by providing basic concepts and practical applications. Hopefully, all who read this book will be better able to diagnose and treat their patients with a MDS.

Harold R. Schumacher, M.D.
Sucha Nand, M.D.

ACKNOWLEDGMENTS

The authors are indebted to a great number of people who have made this book possible.

Secretarial support from Carol Corcoran, Nathalie Geiger, Patricia Hathaway, Regina Rohrkasse, Rose Spencer, and Joyce Turner was invaluable. Without their help, this book would not have been possible.

Pathology residents Drs. Thomas Gilson and Gary Utz were very helpful in supplying articles and reviewing some of the manuscript. Special gratitude is due to my fellows, Drs. Patricia Miller-Canfield, Thomas Debowski, Anwar Mikhael, Charles Stephens, and Achmad Wibowo, who supplied me with numerous articles from the library and read the majority of the manuscript. We further want to thank students Sayana Rajasekhar and Chirag Shah for carefully checking all references in the book.

Excellent photographic support was provided by Jay Card.

Additional appreciation is extended to technologists Cindy Blakemore, Kathleen Comer, Marge Gryzbac, James Hill, Gerardo Perrotta, and Jo Anne Reisinger for their expert technical assistance and advice and for processing all the peripheral blood and bone marrow specimens that are illustrated.

We are indebted to Dr. Raoul Fresco for his critical review of Chapter 5 and for supplying the electron micrographs.

We are greatly indebted to Dr. Paul Hurtubise, who edited Chapter 6, and to Dr. Ken Foon, who provided some of the illustrations for the chapter. Dr. Wendy Stock kindly reviewed Chapter 9.

A very special debt of gratitude to Dr. Michelle Le Beau, who edited Chapter 7 and provided many of the illustrations. Further thanks are due to Dr. Ashok Srivastava for supplying some illustrations for this chapter.

A note of appreciation to Drs. David Askew and Paul Steele for reviewing Chapter 8.

The authors sincerely appreciate the above contributions. They have helped greatly to improve the quality of this book.

FOREWORD

It is a daunting task to undertake the compilation, review, synthesis, and critique of even a limited area of medicine today because of the explosion of knowledge and the complexity of investigative techniques that have developed in the past one to two decades. There has also been an expansion of interest and research in many countries worldwide and publication in languages other than English, which adds further difficulty to keeping current. The subject of myelodysplastic syndromes is complex and confusing. Drs. Schumacher and Nand have undertaken this difficult task and succeeded admirably in organizing and presenting a book which reviews the current state of knowledge of myelodysplastic disorders.

Having had the perspective of working in this field and participating in my own prospective studies, as well as cooperative international studies involving morphological classification, cytogenetic studies, and molecular biology for nearly 30 years, I have seen the evolution of classification, laboratory studies, and therapy.

Although the French-American-British group introduced a classification that has served as a framework of discussion and brought some order out of chaos in this area, there are still many patients who do not fit the classification, and there are areas of the classification that need change or refinement.

Chapter 1 gives a good overview of the development of the concepts of preleukemia and myelodysplasia, and gives credit to the early Italian workers for the initial development of the concept. Although the FAB group, in their initial articles, felt strongly that myelodysplastic processes were not preleukemias, the differences between the concepts are diminishing as we find that the myelodysplastic syndromes share common features with the preleukemias or overt leukemias beyond the morphological findings.

With the perspective of long-term follow-up studies, we learned that our definitions of myelodysplasia and acute leukemia had to be refined. In the early 1960s, those of us who were studying patients with suspected preleukemias were often told by respected clinicians and hematopathologists that there was no such disease. We now recognize that this group of disorders is more common in the population than the overt acute leukemias and that it is a major health problem in older patients.

In Chapter 2, the clinical and morphological features that lead the clinician to suspect the disorder and the pathologist or hematologist to confirm the diagnosis are well covered. The role of abnormal localization of immature precursors (ALIP) in the diagnosis of myelodysplastic syndrome (MDS) and their prognostic significance is discussed. The biopsy features of MDS are of great interest to pathologists who must rely predominantly on the bone marrow biopsy specimen for diagnosis because of lack of access to the bone marrow aspirate.

The scoring systems for prognosis are discussed in Chapter 2. Several scoring systems give good estimates of survival. Great efforts to develop scoring systems hardly seem more than an academic exercise as long as we have no effective means of altering the course of the disease. A prognostic system based on findings that would identify the patient who will transform to acute leukemia and give a reliable estimate of the immediacy of the transformation would have greater clinical value. The greater problem is the accurate identification of MDS patients who present with cytopenias without an increase in blasts.

Chapter 3 addresses the problem of differential diagnosis. The important features that permit differentiation of secondary MDS, aplastic anemia, atypical chronic myeloproliferative disorders, and hereditary disorders that mimic MDS from primary MDS are well presented. The authors discuss the role of cell marker studies in MDS, including cytochemistry and immunocytochemistry in Chapter 4.

Chapter 5 gives a description of electron microscopy in the diagnosis and differential diagnosis of MDS. The use of electron microscopy is limited in these disorders, but in selected cases it can provide important information.

Chapter 6 deals with immunophenotype and immunological abnormalities. The use of immunophenotyping of cells has led to more accurate classification of the MDSs, especially of megakaryocytic involvement and of the types of blasts observed in bone marrows of patients with refractory anemia with excess blasts (RAEB).

Chapter 7 is devoted to the role of cytogenetics in the diagnosis and classification of MDS and leukemia. Cytogenetic studies have been perhaps the most useful laboratory tool in the study of MDS and have contributed greatly to our understanding of the disorder. The practical use of cytogenetic studies in classifying MDS and determining the prognosis are well covered.

Chapter 8 discusses molecular genetic abnormalities in MDS. Ultimately, the answer to the cause and pathogenesis of MDS must depend on alterations in essential cellular mechanisms which control and regulate cell growth and differentiation. A discussion of the techniques used to establish clonality such as G6PD isoenzymes, restriction fragment length polymorphism, studies of X chromosome genes such as phosphoglycerate kinase and hypoxanthine phosphoribosyl transferase combined with X chromosome methylation studies, *RAS* mutations, *FMS* mutations and deletions, and tumor-suppressor genes is given. This chapter gives us a sense of direction where research in MDS is going, but the answers to the enigma of the cause and progression of this group of diseases awaits future studies.

Chapter 9 deals with the clinical features, prognosis, and treatment of MDS. It provides an excellent review of the studies and parameters used in establishing the prognosis. The presence of increased blasts and the severity of neutropenia or thrombocytopenia appear to be the best indicators of survival. Dr. Nand has reviewed this difficult area of treatment and placed the use of various agents in perspective. He points out that patients with advanced forms of the disease with increased blasts, who are behaving like acute leukemias, should be treated as having acute leukemias. If the patient is young, bone marrow transplant should be strongly considered. Erythropoietin, granulocyte—colony stimulating factor, and granulocyte-macrophage colony-stimulating factor may be used to advantage to increase erythroid values and neutrophil counts in an attempt to decrease transfusion requirements and infectious episodes. He also suggests that other maturation agents and cytokines should be used in protocol settings. This chapter gives an excellent approach to the management and therapy of MDS and points out the necessity to develop new therapeutic approaches.

The use of case studies is an effective means of putting all of this knowledge together for the reader, illustrating the diagnostic approach; the use of laboratory tools for diagnosis, classification, and prognosis; and the clinical management of this group of perplexing illnesses.

Drs. Schumacher and Nand have made a significant contribution by developing this text, which presents a comprehensive but easily assimilated overview of a complex and difficult area of a hematologic disease useful both to the practicing clinician and the pathologist.

Robert V. Pierre
Professor of Pathology
University of Southern California
Los Angeles, California

CONTENTS

CHAPTERS

HCK	Hemopoietic cell kinase
HCT	Hematocrit
HGB	Hemoglobin
HIV	Human immunodeficiency virus
HLA	Human leukocyte antigen
HMBA	Hexamethylene bisacetamide
HPRT	Hypoxanthine phosphoribosyl transferase
HTLV	Human T-cell leukemia virus
IFN	Interferon
IL	Interleukin
IRF	Interferon regulatory factor
LAK	Lymphokine activated killer
LAP	Leukocyte alkaline phosphatase
LCA	Leukocyte common antigen
LDH	Lactose dehydrogenase
LGL	Large granular lymphocyte
LHC	Epidermal Langerhans cells
M-CSF	Macrophage colony-stimulating factor
MDR	Multidrug resistance
MAKA	Major karyotypic aberrations
MCH	Mean corpuscular hemoglobin
MCHC	Mean corpuscular hemoglobin concentration
MCV	Mean corpuscular volume
MDS	Myelodysplastic syndrome
MHC	Major histocompatibility complex
MIC	Morphologic, Immunologic, Cytogenetic Cooperative Study Group
MIKA	Minor karyotypic aberrations
MMM	Myelofibrosis with myeloid metaplasia
MoAb	Monoclonal antibody
MPD	Myeloproliferative disorder
MPEX	Myeloperoxidase
MPV	Mean platelet volume
NAP	Neutrophil attractant-activation protein
NF-1	Neurofibromatosis type 1
NF-1	Neurofibromatosis gene
NK	Natural killer
NSE	Nonspecific esterases
PAS	Periodic acid——Schiff
PCR	Polymerase chain reaction
PDGF	Platelet-derived growth factor
PDGFR	Platelet-derived growth factor receptor
PDW	Platelet distribution width
PGK	Phosphoglycerate kinase
Ph^1	Philadelphia chromosome
PK	Pyruvate kinase
PMN	Polymorphonuclear cells
PNH	Paroxysmal nocturnal hemoglobinuria

PPO	Platelet peroxidase
Prog.	Progenitor cells
RA	Refractory anemia
RAEB	Refractory anemia with excess blasts
RAEB-IT	Refractory anemia with excess blasts in transformation
RARS	Refractory anemia with ringed sideroblasts
RBC	Red blood count
RDW	Red cell distribution width
RFLP	Restriction fragment length polymorphisms
RN	Refractory neutropenia
RNA	Ribonucleic acid
RT	Refractory thrombocytopenia
SBB	Sudan black B
t-AML	Therapy-related AML
Th	T-helper
t-MDS	Therapy-related MDS
Tdt	Terminal deoxynucleotidyl transferase
TEM	Transmission electron microscopy
WBC	White blood count

Overview

The myelodysplastic syndromes (MDSs) are a group of clonal proliferative bone marrow disorders resulting in dysmyelopoiesis and peripheral blood cytopenias. These effects have been related to the clonal expansion of a multipotent stem cell. Therefore, by their very essence, the MDSs prior to 1982 created a bewildering nosological array of terms which understandably caused much confusion and consternation. However, in 1982, the FAB Cooperative Groups introduced the term myelodysplastic syndromes for the following five groups that we use today: *refractory anemia (RA), refractory anemia with ringed sideroblasts (RARS), refractory anemia with excess blasts (RAEB), refractory anemia with excess blasts in transformation (RAEB-IT), and chronic myelomonocytic leukemia (CMML)*. Many observers have used *chronic myelomonocytic leukemia in transformation (CMML-IT)* and *myelodysplastic syndrome, unclassified*, to categorize cases not classifiable by FAB MDS criteria.

The diagnosis of a MDS must be made in the appropriate clinical setting and is heavily dependent upon morphology. The hematologist/hematopathologist must be able to identify dyserythropoiesis, dysgranulopoiesis, and dysmegakaryopoiesis within the peripheral blood and bone marrow. Similarly to the staging criteria in chronic lymphocytic leukemia, many investigators have created scoring systems based primarily on levels of hemoglobin, neutrophils, platelets, and bone marrow blasts. One system, which uses a multivariate proportional hazard analysis, includes bone marrow blast percentage, hemoglobin concentration, platelet count, and age. This scoring system seems to define more clearly those patients with variable numbers of bone marrow blasts. Most of the scoring systems are relatively simple to apply in routine clinical practice.

The diagnosis of MDSs can at times be most difficult; therefore, the differential diagnosis is extensive. Acquired disorders such as aplastic anemia, autoimmune and immune disorders (e.g., AIDS), drugs, inflammatory diseases, and inherited disorders such as Fanconi's anemia, Bloom's syndrome, Wiskott-Aldrich syndrome, and others may manifest features that mimic the MDSs. Additionally, since secondary or therapy-related MDS (t-MDS) has created unique diagnostic problems, the Morphologic, Immunologic, Cytogenetic Cooperative Study Group (MIC) added t-MDS to the FAB classification.

Cytochemical stains in general do not have the same impact on the diagnosis as in the acute leukemias. Nevertheless, they are used in a similar manner if the MDS progresses to acute leukemia. By contrast, Prussian blue stain for iron for evaluation of ringed sideroblasts is necessary in all cases. Finally, immunocytochemistry has become increasingly important to evaluate abnormal localization of immature precursors (ALIP), allowing greater insights into the evolution of the myelodysplastic process.

Transmission electron microscopy has rarely been used in the evaluation of MDSs. However, it may be of benefit in extremely difficult cases similar to rare acute and chronic leukemias (especially in helping to determine the origin of blast cells which cannot be clearly classified by other techniques).

Although flow cytometric analysis is not useful in MDSs due to the scarcity of sufficient cells, immunocytochemistry has been used to characterize immature lymphoid, myeloid, erythroid, and megakaryocytic cells. Also, CD34, an early marker of stem cell–myeloid differentiation, has been utilized by some investigators in the initial assessment of MDS patients. Besides immunophenotypic cellular variation in the MDSs, a wide range of immunological abnormalities is present in MDS patients that are poorly understood. These are currently under investigation and will undoubtedly require much greater understanding if we are to treat these disorders effectively.

Cytogenetic analysis appears to be extremely important in the appraisal of the MDSs. Approximately 60% of patients with primary MDSs and 86% of those with t-MDS have abnormal karyotypes. Those with primary MDSs usually have a single numeric change or a structural abnormality involving only one chromosome. Also, some patients may have translocations involving only two chromosomes. By contrast, t-MDSs tend to show multiple chromosomal abnormalities that almost always involve abnormalities of chromosomes 5 and/or 7, alone or in combination. Therefore, karyotypic analysis helps in the differential diagnosis, especially in distinguishing primary MDSs from t-MDSs. Specifically, karyotypic analysis has been most helpful in differentiating hypoplastic MDS from aplastic anemia.

Molecular genetics has greatly increased our understanding of the MDSs. Mutations and/or deletions of the *RAS* family genes, *FMS* gene, and *MPL* gene in the MDSs have begun to offer new insights into the molecular mechanisms underlying the dysplastic process. Furthermore, the finding of deletions of tumor-suppressor genes in MDSs such as p53, the deleted in colorectal carcinoma (*DCC*) gene, and the interferon regulatory factor (*IRF*-1) gene have added new knowledge to this most complex enigma. Also recently, the neurofibromatosis type 1 (*NF1*) gene has been implicated in the origin of the MDSs in early childhood. Rarely, analysis of these genes has been used in the diagnosis of difficult cases.

Besides considering the diagnosis of MDS, this volume addresses its treatment.

Although blood and platelet transfusions, iron chelation, and antibiotics remain the mainstay of therapy, our limited understanding of the pathogenesis of the MDSs contributes to the lack of specificity and effectiveness of our therapeutic interventions. Hematopoietic growth factors, used alone or in combination, may improve the quality of life and survival in some patients, but for the most part they have not been contributory. Even though antileukemic therapy and bone marrow transplantation have a major role in the management of patients younger than 50 years of age, they are not available to the majority of patients who are over 50 years of age.

Like its sister volumes *Acute Leukemia* and *Chronic Leukemia: Approach to Diagnosis*, this book utilizes a multifaceted, unified approach to diagnosis and includes practical cases to reinforce diagnostic concepts. In addition, a chapter on therapy is included to present current information in this most difficult area. Although our understanding of leukemogenesis is still clouded, the MDSs have given us molecular stepping stones in our quest to understand the leukemic process.

CHAPTER 1
Diagnostic Approach

BACKGROUND

Myelodysplastic syndrome (MDS) is a term for a group of clonal proliferative bone marrow disorders which is the result of trilineage dyspoiesis from clonal expansion of a multipotent stem cell resulting in dysmyelopoiesis and peripheral blood cytopenias. This concept was first suggested by Dacie et al. (1959), who noted a dimorphic population of red cells consistent with a clonal disorder. Prior to the widespread use of the term *myelodysplastic syndrome*, hematologists and hematopathologists were burdened with an overwhelming number of confusing terms, including *preleukemia, acute leukemia, subacute myeloid leukemia, smoldering acute leukemia, hemopoietic dysplasia, herald state of leukemia, preleukemic anemia, refractory dysmyelopoietic anemia, dysmyelopoietic syndrome, preleukemia/myelodysplastic syndrome, refractory anemia with excess blasts, refractory anemia, sideroblastic anemia,* and *myeloid dysplasia.* No wonder such confusion reigned.

As early as 1912 and 1917, Copelli and DiGuglielmo, Italian hematologists, recognized that leukemia was not exclusively a white cell disease. Also, DiGuglielmo realized that erythroleukemia could terminate in acute myeloid leukemia. Such observations antedated by over half a century our current concept of defects in a multipotent stem cell. In 1949, Hamilton-Patterson described three adult patients with anemia prior to the onset of acute leukemia. He believed that the anemia was part of the leukemic process and used the term *preleukemic anemia.* Shortly thereafter, the term *preleukemia* was introduced by Block et al. (1953) in an article often credited with introducing the idea that such disorders were a

Table 1.1 Classification of the Myelodysplastic Syndromes

FAB classification
  Refractory anemia (RA)
  Refractory anemia with ringed sideroblasts (RARS)
  Refractory anemia with excess blasts (RAEB)
  Chronic myelomonocytic leukemia (CMML)
  Refractory anemia with excess blasts in transformation (RAEB-IT)
Additional categories
  Chronic myelomonocytic leukemia in transformation (CMML-IT)
  Myelodysplastic syndrome, unclassified

harbinger of acute leukemia. Eleven of 12 patients reported developed acute leukemia, and Block and co-workers expanded the concept of preleukemia to encompass cytopenias of all lineages. Therefore, by midcentury, the relationship between the idiopathic cytopenias and the subsequent onset of acute myelogenous leukemia had become broadly appreciated. In 1960, Vilter and associates described five types of refractory anemia with hypercellular marrow. Their type 3 appeared to be refractory anemia with excess blasts (RAEB), included in the current French-American-British (FAB) classification. Three of five such patients died of acute leukemia. In 1974, Linman and Saarni firmly established the term *preleukemia* in the literature and emphasized the multilineage marrow dyspoiesis in these disorders. In 1976, the FAB Cooperative Group presented their landmark article on the classification of the acute leukemias. In this article, they separated two broad types of dysmyelopoietic syndrome: RAEB and chronic myelomonocytic leukemia (CMML). They cautioned that an immediate recommendation to start therapy cannot be made or may not be indicated in these two disorders. Further, they commented that frequent follow-up of peripheral blood counts and repeated bone marrow examinations to check for possible progression toward acute myeloid leukemia was indicated. RAEB and CMML were designated *dysmyelopoietic syndromes (DMPS)*. In 1982, the FAB Cooperative Group abandoned this term in favor of the now popular term *myelodysplastic syndrome*. At that time, they included three new subsets of (or for) this disorder: refractory anemia (RA), RA with ringed sideroblasts (RARS), and RAEB in transformation (RAEB-IT). The FAB classification of the MDSs is presented in Table 1.1. CMML in transformation (CMML-IT) and unclassified MDS are two additional categories used by many observers for those cases of MDS that cannot be classified by FAB criteria.

CELL BIOLOGY OF MDSs

The essential features of MDSs are ineffective bone marrow maturation and insufficient release of leukocytes, erythrocytes, and platelets or permutations of these elements into the peripheral blood. The indispensable morphological features are manifested as dyserythropoiesis, dysgranulopoiesis, and dysmegakaryocytopoiesis; the result is maturation arrest within the marrow and cytopenias within the peripheral blood. These abnormal morphological findings in MDS are often

Table 1.2   Some of the Common Oncogenes and Anti-Oncogenes Implicated in the MDSs

Oncogene Anti-oncogene	Chromosome	Gene Product (kd)	Biochemical Activity	Function	Site
NRAS	1p11–13	21	GTPase	Signal transduction	Cytoplasm
HRAS	11p14–15	21	GTPase	Signal transduction	Cytoplasm
KRAS	12p12	21	GTPase	Signal transduction	Cytoplasm
FMS	5q34	140	Tyrosine kinase	M-CSF receptor*	Membrane
p53	17p13	53	—	Tumor suppressor	Nucleus
IRF-1	5q31.1	38–40	Transcriptional activator	Tumor suppressor	Nucleus

*M-CSF = macrophage colony-stimulating factor.

described as clonal hemopathies because they originate from malignant clones derived from a single abnormal hematopoietic stem cell. Therefore, normal hematopoiesis is polyclonal, controlled, and regulated; however, hematopoiesis of MDS is monoclonal, uncontrolled, and not appropriately regulated.

These abnormal hematopoietic clones have been recognized in patients with MDS by means of cytogenetic, glucose-6-phosphate dehydrogenase (G6PD), restriction fragment length polymorphisms (RFLP), and polymerase chain reaction (PCR) studies. The latter three techniques have the advantage of detecting abnormal clones without any recognizable karyotypic abnormalities. Cytogenetic analyses have demonstrated that karyotypic abnormalities are present in about 50% of patients with MDS. G6PD isoenzyme analysis and RFLP detect clonality of abnormal hematopoiesis based on the Lyon hypothesis that only one X chromosome is active in each female cell. Therefore, monoclonal cell proliferations can be detected when cells express the same G6PD enzyme variant from females heterozygous at the G6PD locus. The RFLP technique uses the principle that maternal and paternal copies of the X chromosomes can be detected in female cells at the DNA level by analyzing RFLP. Since gene activation is associated with changes in the methylation of cytosine residues, the active X chromosome, either maternal or paternal, can be detected as clonal in MDS. Apparently, the RFLP stategy can detect tumor clonality in a greater number of females than can G6PD isoenzyme testing. PCR has the advantage of detecting a small abnormal clone within the background of normal cells by using selective oligonucleotide hybridization to mutated somatic genes.

Since MDSs are strikingly heterogeneous in their clinical phenotypes, there is an ever-increasing number of observations concerning chromosomal abnormalities, mutated cellular proto-oncogenes, and altered production of hematopoietic growth factors. Some of the oncogenes and anti-oncogenes implicated in MDSs are shown in Table 1.2. The interactions of these various factors are enormously complicated, and we have just begun to deal with this most difficult hematopoietic conundrum. There is no unifying hypothesis which allows us to begin to explain what we observe in our patients. Nevertheless, Yoshida (1993) has hypothesized that apoptosis may be the mechanism responsible for the premature intramedullary cell death in the MDSs. However, he adds that although no formal proof of apoptosis occurring in vivo in MDS marrow has been presented, MDS cells may be unusually susceptible to apoptosis, due probably to genetic instability and impaired maturation.

Table 1.3   Diagnostic Approach to MDS

Pertinent clinical data
Peripheral smear
Complete hemogram*
Morphology of bone marrow: aspirate, touch preparations, biopsy, and clot
Cytochemistry and terminal deoxynucleotidyl transferase
Immunophenotype by flow cytometry
Immunocytochemistry
Cytogenetics and interphase analysis†
Electron microscopy‡
Gene rearrangement analysis‡
Oncogene analysis‡
Tissue culture‡
Polymerase chain reaction‡
Miscellaneous: analysis of defective granulocyte and platelet function; evaluation of
    hemoglobin, especially F; testing for red blood cell abnormalities, paroxysmal
    nocturnal hemoglobinuria, red cell inclusion (hemoglobin H), phosphokinase
    deficiency, and blood group changes; blood and urine muramidase, testing for HIV,
    serum folate, vitamin B_{12}

*Includes differential count, WBC, RBC, HCT, HGB, MCV, MCH, MCHC, red cell distribution width
(RDW), mean platelet volume (MPV), platelet distribution width (PDW), reticulocyte, and platelet
counts.
†Especially to demonstrate chromosomal changes which equate with the prognosis.
‡Special cases.

The aberrant products or lack of products produced by the various oncogenes and/or anti-oncogenes might be likened to a symphony orchestra that creates a cacophony of disharmonious sounds. Deletions of the long arms of chromosomes 5 and 7; deletion of tissue plasminogen activator inhibitor and the multidrug resistance (*MDR*) genes; mutations involving c-*FMS* in chronic myelomonocytic leukemia; activation of *RAS* oncogenes by point mutations; and autocrine production of granulocyte-macrophage colony-stimulating factor (GM-CSF) and interleukin-6 (IL-6) in CMML are but a few of the diverse abnormalities observed in MDS. Recently, the interferon regulatory factor-1 (IRF-1), characterized by anti-oncogene activity, was discovered to be encoded by a gene mapped to 5q31.1. Interestingly, this gene was consistently deleted at one or both alleles in nine cases of acute leukemia and four cases of MDS. Therefore, IRF-1 may be an important deleted gene in human leukemia and myelodysplasias. Also, the deleted in colorectal carcinoma (*DCC*) gene and the type 1 neurofibromatosis (*NF*-1) gene have been recently implicated in the MDSs.

DIAGNOSIS: THE APPROACH

Diagnosis of the MDSs, like that of the acute and chronic leukemias, requires a unified, multifaceted approach. The diagnosis should be strongly entertained in the setting of neutropenia, thrombocytopenia, unexplained anemia, and/or monocytosis in an older patient without the usual explanations of marrow failure. The diagnostic approach used to establish a diagnosis is presented in Table 1.3.

The approach is similar to that used in the acute leukemias since the evolution of these disorders frequently terminates in acute leukemia. In this time of cost containment, it should be emphasized that the diagnosis can be established with a minimum number of studies, with examination of the peripheral blood smear, bone marrow aspirate, bone marrow biopsy, cytohistochemistries, and cytogenetics being adequate in most cases. Also, Prussian blue stain for iron, preferably on the aspirate, and reticulin for fibrosis on the biopsy specimen are indicated. Again, as stated in our previous books on acute and chronic leukemias, adequate sample material must be obtained and technical procedures must be of the highest quality. The most simple diagnosis may be missed because of inadequate sampling and poor technical quality of the material—the principal cause of misdiagnosis.

SUMMARY

Excellent peripheral blood and bone marrow specimens demonstrating good morphology combined with cytohistochemistry (including Prussian blue stain for iron and reticulin stains) remains the gold standard of diagnosis in the MDSs. Already, the newer technologies have begun to have an impact on our diagnostic capabilities. Flow cytometric analysis, interphase cytogenetic testing, oncogene examination by Southern blot and PCR methodology have started to influence both diagnosis and treatment, especially with regard to minimal residual disease. We have only begun to understand the complexities of the leukemias and the MDSs. With increased comprehension, better diagnostic techniques will be developed.

BIBLIOGRAPHY

Articles

Block M, Jacobson LO, Bethard WF: Preleukemic human leukemia. *JAMA* 152:1018–1028, 1953.

Copelli M: Di una emopatia sistemizzata cappresentata da una iperplasia eritroblastica (erithromatosi). *Pathologica* 4:460–465, 1912.

Dacie JV, Smith MD, White JC, et al: Refractory normoblastic anaemia: A clinical and haematological study of seven cases. *Br J Haematol* 5:56–82, 1959.

DiGuglielmo G: *Le Malattie Eritremiche ed Eritroleucemiche.* Rome, II Pensiero Scientifico Editore, 1962.

DiGuglielmo G: Ricerche di ematologia. *Folia Med* 13:386–396, 1917.

DiGuglielmo G: Le Eritremie. *Haematologica* 9:301–312, 1928.

Geddes AD, Bowen DT, Jacobs A: Clonal karyotype abnormalities and clinical progress in the myelodysplastic syndrome. *Br J Haematol* 76:194–202, 1990.

Hamilton-Patterson JL: Preleukemic anaemia. *Acta Haematol* 2:309–316, 1949.

Janssen JWG, Buschle M, Layton M, et al: Clonal analysis of myelodysplastic syndromes: Evidence of a multipotent stem cell origin. *Blood* 73:248–254, 1989.

Kerkhofs H, Hermans J, Haak HL, et al: Utility of the FAB classification for myelodysplastic syndromes: Investigation of prognostic factors in 237 cases. *Br J Haematol* 65:73–81, 1987.

Linman JW, Saarni MI: The preleukemic syndrome. *Semin Hematol* 11:93–100, 1974.

Miyoke K, Inokuchi K, Dan K, et al: Alterations in the deleted colorectal carcinoma gene in human primary leukemia. *Blood* 82:927–930, 1993a.

Miyoke K, Inokuchi K, Dan K, et al: Expression of the DCC gene in myelodysplastic syndromes and overt leukemia. *Leuk Res* 17:755–788, 1993b.

Pierre RV, Catovsky D, Mufti GJ, et al: Clinical–cytogenetic correlations in myelodysplasia (preleukemia). *Cancer Genet Cytogenet* 40:149–161, 1989.

Shannon KM, O'Connell P, Martin GA, et al: Loss of normal NF-1 allele from the bone marrow of children with type 1 neurofibromatosis and malignant myeloid disorders. *N Engl J Med* 330:597–601, 1994.

Suciu S, Kuse R, Weh HJ, et al: Results of chromosome studies and their relation to morphology, course, and prognosis in 120 patients with de novo myelodysplastic syndrome. *Cancer Genet Cytogenet* 44:15–26, 1990.

Vilter RW, Jarrod T, Will JJ, et al: Refractory anemia with hyperplastic bone marrow. *Blood* 15:1–29, 1960.

Vogelstein B, Fearon ER, Hamilton SR, et al: Clonal analysis using recombinant DNA probes from the X-chromosome. *Cancer Res* 47:4806–4813, 1987.

Willman CL, Sever CE, Pollavicini MG, et al: Deletion of IRF-1, mapping to chromosome 5q31.1, in human leukemia and preleukemic myelodysplasia. *Science* 259:968–971, 1993.

Yoshida Y: Hypothesis: Apoptosis may be the mechanism responsible for the premature intramedullary cell death in myelodysplastic syndrome. *Leukemia* 7:144–146, 1993.

Yunis JJ, Lobell M, Arnesen MA, et al: Refined chromosome study helps define prognostic subgroups in most patients with primary myelodysplastic syndrome and acute myelogenous leukaemia. *Br J Hematol* 68:189–194, 1988.

Review Articles

Bennett JM, Catovsky D, Daniel MT, et al: Proposals for the classification of the acute leukemias (FAB cooperative group). *Br J Haematol* 33:451–458, 1976.

Bennett JM, Catovsky D, Daniel MT, et al: Proposals for the classification of the myelodysplastic syndromes (FAB cooperative group). *Br J Haematol* 51:189–199, 1982.

Beris P: Primary clonal myelodysplastic syndromes. *Semin Hematol* 26:216–233, 1989.

Cline MJ: Mechanisms of disease: The molecular basis of leukemia. *N Engl J Med* 330:328–336, 1994.

Greenberger JS: The hematopoietic microenvironment. *Crit Rev Oncol Hematol* 11:65–84, 1991.

Koeffler HP: Myelodysplastic syndromes. Hematol Oncol Clin North Am, Philadelphia, 1992, pp 1–728.

Noël P, Solberg LA: Myelodysplastic syndromes: Pathogenesis, diagnosis, and treatment. *Crit Rev Oncol/Hematol* 12:193–215, 1992.

Pierre RV: Preleukemic/myelodysplasia. *Curr Hematol Oncol* 6:131–162, 1988.

CHAPTER 2
Morphology, Classification, and Scoring

GENERAL COMMENTS

In order to accurately diagnose, classify, and score the MDSs, high-quality Wright-Giemsa or Romanowsky stains of the peripheral blood, bone marrow aspirate, and touch preparations of bone marrow biopsy are absolutely essential. Clot and biopsy material should be placed in B5 fixative solution and the biopsy decalcified, embedded in paraffin, cut at 4 μm, and stained with hematoxylin and eosin. The appropriate clinical setting combined with unexplained anemia, neutropenia, thrombocytopenia, and/or monocytosis without a suitable explanation should alert the hematologist and hematopathologist to the possibility of an MDS. This suspicion is further upheld by the findings of dyserythropoiesis, dysgranulopoiesis, or dysmegakaryopoiesis within the peripheral blood and bone marrow. Although these peripheral blood findings may arouse great suspicion of a MDS, bone marrow examination is absolutely essential for diagnosis. In addition to the standard cytochemical and histochemical stains mentioned above, Prussian blue stain for iron, reticulin stain for fibrosis, and, rarely, silver stain for ringed sideroblasts in iron-deficient patients should be employed. These and other cytochemical stains (peroxidase, Sudan black B, and combined esterase) will be addressed in detail in Chapter 4.

The diagnosis, although heavily dependent on morphology, should be multifaceted, systematic, and thorough to firmly establish the correct diagnosis. One should always be sure that all necessary material is obtained prior to treatment, since institution of therapy will irrevocably alter subsequent analysis of material.

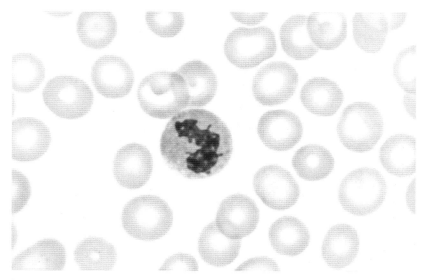

Figure 2.4 Peripheral blood from the patient in Fig. 2.3 demonstrating numerous nuclear sticks (×1,000).

been seen in both MDSs and MPDs. In one series, ringed granulocytic nuclei were present in 25% of the cases. Nuclear sticks may be observed in some cases of primary MDS, but are more common in therapy-related MDS (t-MDS) (Fig. 2.4).

Of the granular abnormalities, hypogranulation is most commonly seen, and the more immature forms are often devoid of all granules (Fig. 2.5). The hypogranular cells can be associated with a negative peroxidase staining reaction. Occasion-

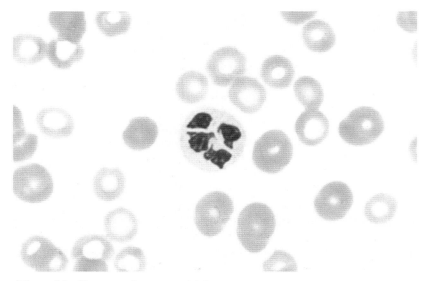

Figure 2.5 Hypogranular neutrophil from a patient with RAEB-IT. PB (×1,000).

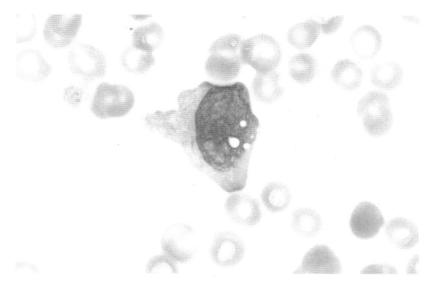

Figure 2.6   Blast cell with an Auer rod and nuclear vacuolization from a patient with RAEB-IT. PB (×1,000).

ally, persistent cytoplasmic basophilia and excess granulation may be seen. Rarely, giant granules similar to those in the Chediak-Higashi syndrome have been reported. Circulating blast cells are frequently observed in RAEB and RAEB-IT (Fig. 2.6).

Since dysgranulopoiesis is the predominant finding in the MDSs, infection is the most common cause of death. In addition to the above-mentioned morphological abnormalities, impaired microbicidal capacity, as well as decreased phagocytic adhesion and chemotaxis, have been reported. Although physiological impairment exists, no correlation has been demonstrated between the risk of infection and the degree of hypogranulation.

Platelet Abnormalities

Thrombocytopenia is common in MDS, and large hypogranular and/or hypergranular platelets can be observed (Fig. 2.7). Thrombocytosis can be seen in the 5q- syndrome and RARS. On electron microscopy, microtubular disorganization, vacuolization, and a dilated canalicular system are seen. Numerous platelet abnormalities have been noted, including platelet peroxidase deficiency, adhesion and aggregation defects, and the presence of surface immunoproteins. The last tend to occur in much higher concentration than those seen in immune thrombocytopenia and may reflect nonspecific binding. Berndt et al. (1988) have reported an acquired Bernard-Soulier-like platelet defect associated with juvenile MDS and monosomy 7.

Overt bleeding tends to be associated with severe thrombocytopenia. These platelet abnormalities can be accompanied by a tendency toward bleeding despite normal platelet counts. Also, abnormal bleeding times have been frequently correlated with a dense-granule storage pool defect.

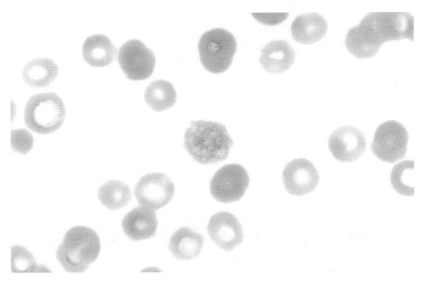

Figure 2.7 Peripheral blood from a patient with RAEB blasts revealing a giant hypergranulated platelet (×1,000).

BONE MARROW

Dyserythropoiesis

The bone marrow aspirate, which is used to evaluate primarily qualitative cytological changes, reveals megaloblastoid and megaloblastic maturation, multinuclearity (Fig. 2.8), bizarre nuclear shapes, mitoses, nuclear dyskinesis (Fig. 2.9), abnor-

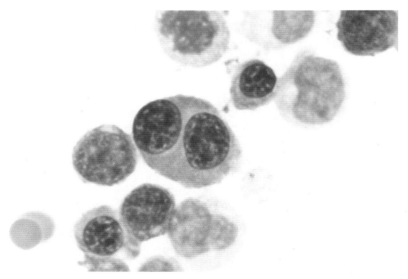

Figure 2.8 Bone marrow from a patient with RAEB-IT showing nucleated red blood cell with two nuclei. Note the megaloblastoid maturation (×1,000).

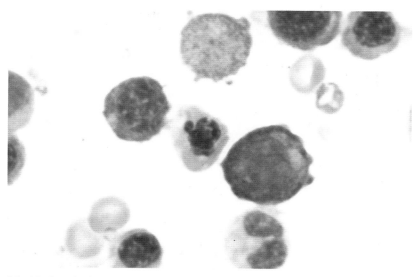

Figure 2.9 Nuclear dyskinesis in a polychromatophilic normoblast (center) from the patient in Fig. 2.8 BM (×1,000).

mally dense chromatin, internuclear bridging, and broad-based nuclear budding. Internuclear bridging has been described in congenital dyserythropoietic anemia type I and may account, in part, for ineffective hematopoiesis. Apparently, internuclear bridging may represent impaired mitosis leading to the deletion and/or addition of chromosomes characteristic of MDS. Cytoplasmic abnormalities include impaired hemoglobinization (ghosted cytoplasm), intense and/or punctate basophilia, cytoplasmic vacuolization, and Howell-Jolly bodies (Fig. 2.10).

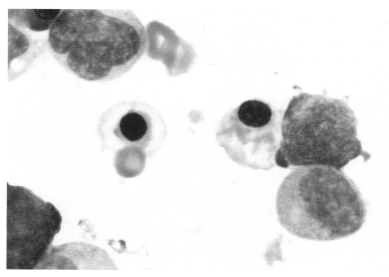

Figure 2.10 One nucleated red blood cell with ghosted cytoplasm (left) and another with vacuolated cytoplasm from a patient with RAEB. BM (×1,000).

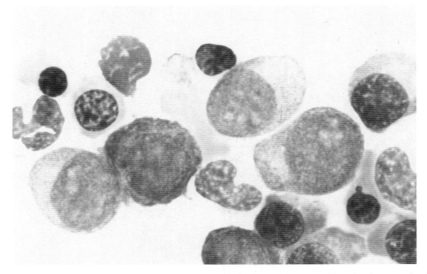

Figure 2.11   Bone marrow from a patient with RAEB-IT showing a type I blast (right center) without granules and a type II blast (upper center) with a few granules. Note proerythroblast (left center) (×1,000).

Prussian blue staining may show the presence of pathological type III sideroblasts, which are defined by some authors as having five or more large granules encircling more than one-third of the nuclear rim. However, slightly more than one-third of the nuclear rim does not constitute a ring. Some authors have even included cases with clusters of five or more ferritin granules not surrounding the nucleus as pathological sideroblasts and have counted them with ring sideroblasts. These sideroblasts are not ringed and perhaps should be classified as pathological type IV sideroblasts. In most cases, the majority of true ringed sideroblasts have five or more granules that encircle at least two-thirds of the nucleus. Only such cells deserve the label *ringed sideroblasts*; however, those not fulfilling such criteria require further descriptive terminology. Quantitative changes in the marrow associated with anemia in the peripheral blood include the presence of more than 15% ringed sideroblasts (expressed as a percentage of all the erythroid nucleated cells) and a proportion of erythroid precursors between 5% and 50%. If the erythroid cells account for more than 50% of the total nucleated cells in the marrow, a diagnosis of erythroleukemia must be considered.

Dysgranulopoiesis

The bone marrow demonstrates left-shifted myeloid maturation, with an increase in type I and type II blasts in appropriate cases of MDS. Type I blasts are myeloblasts of variable size that are devoid of any primary azurophilic granules or Auer rods. Type II blasts were described originally as blasts that may contain a few granules (Fig. 2.11). Initially, the authors used five or fewer granules as a criterion for type II blasts. Currently, we utilize 15 or fewer granules in a cell with features of a myeloblast lacking a Golgi zone as a criterion for a type II blast. We

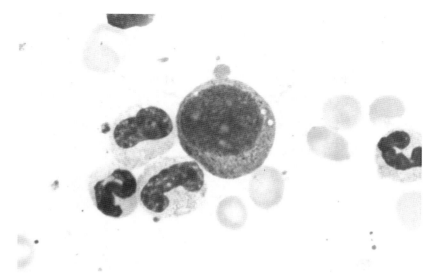

Figure 2.12 Type III blast with multiple nucleoli, immature nuclear structure, more than 20 granules and lacking a Golgi zone in a patient with RAEB and a 5q- karyotype. Note that other granulocytic elements lack granules. BM (×1,000).

have extended this criterion to include monoblasts. Monocytic cells which contain more than 15 granules are designated *promonocytes*. The type III blast, described by Goasguen et al. (1991) as a myeloblast with 20 or more azurophilic granules without a Golgi zone, has not been used by most hematologists and hematopathologists (Fig. 2.12). Obviously, such use would place more MDS patients in the acute leukemia category. This is probably not satisfactory since most MDS patients are elderly and do not tolerate chemotherapy well.

In addition to increased blasts, such abnormalities as pseudo–Pelger-Huët cells, ring-shaped nuclei (Fig. 2.13), hypersegmentation, abnormal or absent staining of the primary and secondary granules, and dense peripheral cytoplasmic basophilia may be observed. Macrophages laden with iron are frequently seen and reflect the underlying ineffective erythropoiesis.

Dysmegakaryopoiesis

Striking morphological changes occur in megakaryocytic precursors in as many as 50% of patients. Large hypolobulated and mononuclear megakaryocytes, megakaryocytes with multiple separate nuclei, and micromegakaryocytes are frequently observed (Fig. 2.14). The micromegakaryocytes ("dwarf forms") commonly reveal multiple small nuclei reminiscent of the polymorphonuclear neutrophils of megaloblastic anemia. These micromegakaryocytes and megakaryoblasts are best identified by using antibodies to platelet glycoproteins. Utilization of an antibody to glycoprotein IIIa has shown that 25% of MDS megakaryocytes are micromegakaryocytes compared to less than 10% in normal marrows. Kuriyama et al. (1986) have observed that micromegakaryocytes in combination with Pelgeroid granulocytes may be the most specific dysplastic marker of MDS. Also, the 5q- syndrome has

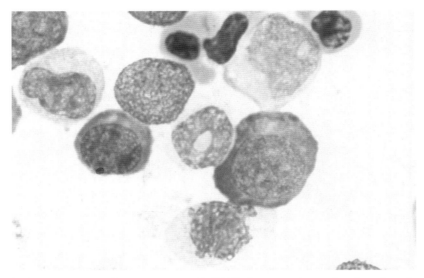

Figure 2.13 Bone marrow from a patient with RAEB demonstrating a ring-shaped nucleus in a granulocytic precursor. Note the nuclear dyskinesis in the polychromatophilic normoblast in the right upper corner (×1,000).

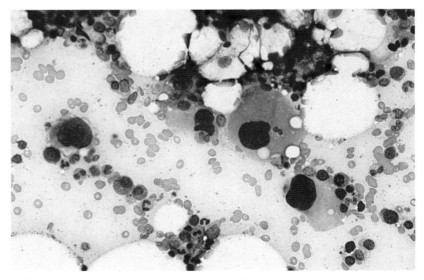

Figure 2.14 Bone marrow showing numerous nonlobulated micromegakaryocytes in a patient with the 5q- syndrome. Note the eccentrically placed nuclei in the majority of these abnormal megakaryocytes (×400).

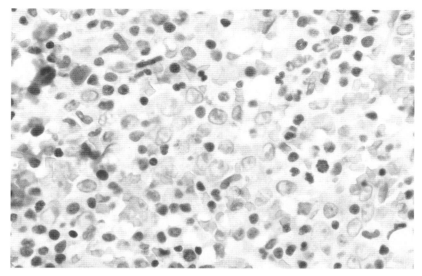

Figure 2.15   Bone marrow biopsy specimen showing ALIP in a patient with RAEB. Note the cluster of light-staining nuclei and prominent nucleoli in the center of the microphotograph (×400).

been associated with a dwarf megakaryocyte with an eccentrically placed small, mononuclear, round nucleus (Fig. 2.14). Since hypogranulation was observed by Wong and Chan (1991) in 80% of their cases of MDS, they have proposed that hypogranulation be included as one of the cytological features of MDS.

Although the qualitative changes noted above are more frequent than quantitative findings, such variations do exist. Even though megakaryocytes are usually normal in number, hypoplasia and hyperplasia can occasionally be observed. Of diagnostic importance is that MDS with megakaryocytic hyperplasia should not be confused with idiopathic thrombocytopenic purpura.

The bone marrow biopsy specimen in MDS is usually hypercellular, although hypocellular specimens may be observed in some patients. The hypocellular variant of MDS, as a separate clinicopathological entity, has been described by one of us (S.N.). This group was characterized by severe cytopenias, a low incidence of leukemic transformation, and unresponsiveness to therapy. Erythroid islands of immature erythroblasts, as well as clusters of immature myeloid cells localized between bony trabeculae, can be seen histologically. These have been referred to as *abnormal localization of immature precursors (ALIP)*.

ABNORMAL LOCALIZATION OF IMMATURE PRECURSORS (ALIP)

The majority of MDS patients demonstrate the presence of ALIP (Fig. 2.15). In normal bone marrows, myeloid precursors are found almost exclusively on the endosteal surface. ALIP have been defined as an accumulation of at least five immature myeloid cells clustering centrally in the bone marrow.

Krause first described ALIP in 1981 and showed that they are of prognostic importance in MDS. Using plastic embedding techniques, Tricot et al. (1984) showed that ALIP were observed in all cases in which the bone marrow aspirate showed greater than 5% blasts. Therefore, the presence of ALIP is important only in cases showing less than 5% blasts on the bone marrow aspirate. Tricot et al. also demonstrated that ALIP-positive patients had a poor survival and a higher risk of leukemic transformation than patients without ALIP. Recently, Lambertenghi-Delilers et al. (1993) evaluated 106 patients with MDS and determined three patterns of bone marrow blastic infiltration: diffuse increase in blasts without aggregation; cluster aggregates of no more than six blasts; and large aggregates of more than six blasts. Diffuse and small-cluster patients had a relatively good prognosis, with median survival of 33 and 46 months, respectively. However, the prognosis in cluster patients with fibrosis was poor (median survival, 14 months). These patients died of bone marrow failure, not of leukemic transformation. By comparison, patients with large clusters without fibrosis showed early leukemic transformation and a poor prognosis (median survival, 12 months).

One major problem with the routine use of ALIP is the inability to identify accurately clusters of immature precursors on trephine biopsy specimens. This problem has been partially overcome by the use of combined cytochemistry and indirect immunoperoxidase techniques, enabling the hematologist and hematopathologist to identify correctly myeloblastic, proerythroblastic, and micromegakaryocytic aggregates. The aggregates of proerythroblasts and micromegakaryocytes are classified as pseudo-ALIP but can look like true ALIP on hematoxylin-eosin or Giemsa stains. Pseudo-ALIP lack a prognosis of malignancy and need to be distinguished from true ALIP, in which clusters of immature cells in the intertrabecular region are of myeloid (granulocytic and monocytic) lineage by cytochemical and immunohistochemical techniques. Mangi and Mufti (1991) have shown that true ALIP are present in all cases of RAEB, RAEB-IT, and CMML with a high peripheral blood cell count. In addition, 14 of 29 (48%) cases of RA and RARS demonstrated the presence of ALIP-like clusters on hematoxylin-eosin and Giemsa staining of the marrow biopsy specimen. However, 8 of the 14 (55%) ALIP were not composed of granulocytic/monocytic aggregates, since they stained for erythroid/megakaryocytic markers. Therefore, bone marrow hypercellularity caused by granulocytic/monocytic hyperplasia is almost always associated with ALIP, whereas approximately half of the cases with ALIP not associated with granulocytic/monocytic hyperplasia (RA/RARS) demonstrate erythroid/megakaryocytic pseudo-ALIP. Furthermore, patients with RA and RARS with granulocytic/monocytic clusters had shorter survivals and an increased incidence of leukemic conversion. These findings are significant in that cases with marked granulocytic hyperplasia correlate with poor survival and a high risk of leukemic transformation. Finally, the ability to divide MDS patients into ALIP+ and ALIP− groups has been highly reproducible.

MYELOFIBROSIS

Myelofibrosis refers to the focal or generalized increase in the number and thickness of reticulin fibers in the bone marrow detected by a silver impregnation stain on

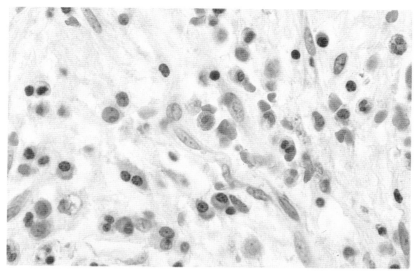

Figure 2.16 Numerous fibroblasts in a bone marrow biopsy specimen from a patient with RA and deletion of chromosome 7 (×400).

a bone marrow biopsy specimen. Approximately half of MDS patients show mild to moderate myelofibrosis, but marked reticulin fibrosis is observed much less frequently (Fig. 2.16).

Islam et al. (1984) have devised a scoring system for changes in the reticulin network in which normal content (grade 0) and four grades of increased bone marrow fibers are distinguished. Some authors consider only grade 3 (combined reticulin and collagen fibers) and grade 4 (predominantly collagen fibers) as significant myelofibrosis.

MDS patients with myelofibrosis have minimal organomegaly, hypercellular marrow with fibrosis, trilineage dysplasia, pancytopenia, and abnormal megakaryocytic proliferation with a predominance of small forms with hypolobulated nuclei. When these features are present, the diagnosis is relatively easy. However, sometimes the distinction between MDS and other myeloproliferative disorders may be difficult. The differential diagnosis includes primary myelofibrosis, accelerated phase of chronic myelogenous leukemia (CML), acute megakaryocytic leukemia (FAB M7), AML with trilineage dysplasia, post-polycythemic myeloid metaplasia, and the rare entity of acute myelofibrosis.

FAB CLASSIFICATION AND DIAGNOSIS

The FAB classification with the diagnostic criteria are shown in Table 2.1. As stated in Chapter 1, additional categories, including MDS, unclassified, and chronic CMML-IT are used by many observers to classify those cases that do not fit into the FAB groups. CMML-IT represents those cases of CMML evolving to the transformation stage. We utilize the FAB criteria for RAEB-IT in establishing

Table 2.1 FAB Classification and Diagnostic Criteria for MDS

Diagnosis	Peripheral Blood	Bone Marrow	Comment
RA	<1% blasts Red cell abnormalities Granulocyte abnormalities Thrombocytopenia Reticulocytopenia	<5% blasts Ringed sideroblasts <15% Dyserythropoiesis Occasional dysgranulopoiesis/dysmegakaryopoiesis	Anemia Refractory cytopenias
RARS	<1% blasts Red cell abnormalities Dimorphic red blood cells Less dysgranulopoiesis	Typically hypercellular <5% blasts Less dysgranulopoiesis and dysmegakaryocytopoiesis >15% ringed sideroblasts	Deficient hemoglobinization Iron within mitochondria
RAEB	<5% blasts Granulocyte abnormalities (more than above) Red cell abnormalities Platelet abnormalities	5–20% blasts (types I and II) Dysplasia of two or more cell lines	Greater progression to acute leukemia than above
CMML	<5% blasts Monocytosis >10^9/L Often increased mature granulocytes, with or without dysgranulopoiesis	Variable trilineage dysplasia (usually) <5% blasts Occasionally 5–20% blasts; may show significant increase in monocytic precursors	Criticized because of poor prognostic power and failure to distinguish from MPD
RAEB-IT	≥5% blasts or more (30% or more is considered acute leukemia by some authors)* Dysgranulopoiesis Unequivocal Auer rod in granulocytic precursors*	*21–30% blasts (Types I and II)	Patients under 50 years of age should be classified as FAB-M2 AML because of treatment response

*Any one of these constitutes a diagnosis of RAEB-IT.

a diagnosis of CMML-IT in a patient with CMML who has evolved or in a patient who fulfills the criteria at diagnosis.

Refractory Anemia (RA)

RA (Fig. 2.17) is usually found in patients over 50 years of age with anemia (hemoglobin less than 11 g/dL) and reticulocytopenia. Rarely, patients without anemia who have neutropenia and/or thrombocytopenia are included in this category. For this reason, some authors have referred to these patients as having *refractory cytopenia*. Also, very rarely, red cell aplasia has been observed in RA patients.

Refractory Anemia with Ringed Sideroblasts (RARS)

RARS, or acquired idiopathic sideroblastic anemia (AISA) (Fig. 2.18), differs from RA by the presence of ringed sideroblasts, which account for more than 15% of

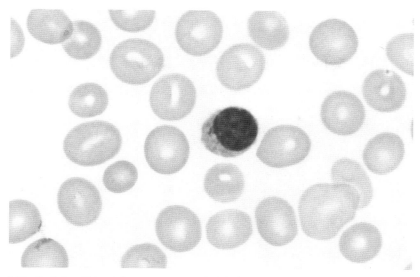

Figure 2.17 Peripheral blood from a patient with RA showing macrocytes. Note the size of the red blood cells in relation to that of the small lymphocyte (×1,000).

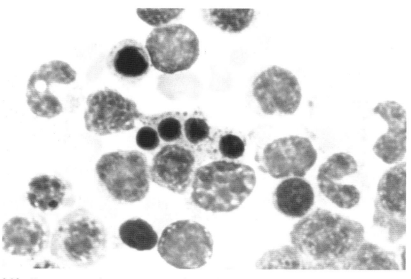

Figure 2.18 Bone marrow from a patient with RARS. Note the dark punctate dots in the cytoplasm of small, pyknotic red cell precursors (center). This most likely represents iron, since iron stain confirmed the presence of ringed sideroblasts (×1,000).

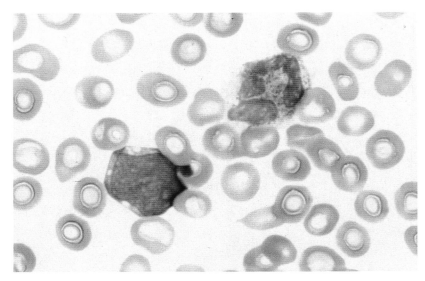

Figure 2.19 Peripheral blood from a patient with RAEB showing a blast cell with nuclear extension and a hypergranulated neutrophil (×1,000).

the nucleated red cell precursors. Type I sideroblasts with one or two granules and type II sideroblasts with five or fewer granules of iron are considered non-pathological and do not ring. Their iron is deposited in siderosomes. Type III ringed sideroblasts, as discussed previously, are pathological and the iron is intramitochondrial in location.

Refractory Anemia with Excess Blasts (RAEB)

The age incidence of RAEB (Fig. 2.19) is similar to that of RA. The dysgranulopoiesis is much more common than in RA. Conspicuous abnormalities are observed in all three cell lines in the peripheral blood. Some cytopenia affecting two or more cell lines is always seen in the peripheral blood. The bone marrow is hypercellular and shows various degrees of either granulocytic or erythrocytic hyperplasia. There is always evidence of dysgranulopoiesis, dyserythropoiesis, or dysmegakaryopoiesis (or combinations). Ringed sideroblasts may be demonstrated. Within the granulocytic series, there is almost always evidence of maturation to promyelocytes and beyond.

Chronic Myelomonocytic Leukemia (CMML)

The defining feature of CMML (Fig. 2.20) is the presence of an absolute monocytosis (>1 × 10^9/L) in the peripheral blood. This is often associated with an increase in mature granulocytes, with or without dysgranulopoiesis. The percentage of blasts in the peripheral blood is less than 5%. Variable degrees of trilineage dysplasia are observed. Typically, less than 5% blasts are found in the marrow, but occasionally the marrow contains 5% to 20% blasts and exhibits features similar to those of RAEB.

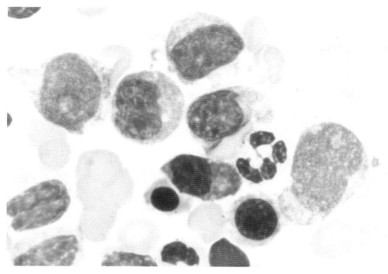

Figure 2.20   Bone marrow from a patient with CMML showing a nest of immature monocytic precursors and blasts. Note the agranular neutrophil (×1,000).

The inclusion of CMML in the classification of MDS has been criticized for two main reasons. Firstly, the classification provides poor prognostic power, as evidenced by the wide range of survival. Although some authors have used Bournemouth scoring in stratifying the prognosis, which has proved to be very predictive of survival in MDS patients in general, it revealed less prognostic value in CMML. This is apparently due to the tendency toward neutrophilia rather than neutropenia.

Secondly, the classification fails to distinguish clearly between CMML and the chronic myeloproliferative disorders. This is best illustrated by a patient who presents with a WBC count of 50 × 10^9/L, 3% blasts and 4% monocytes in the peripheral blood; a hypercellular, moderately dysplastic marrow with 7% blasts and 6% monocytes; and a normal karyotype. This scenario could satisfy the criteria of RAEB, CMML, or Ph[1]-negative CML when evaluated by different observers. This problem could be resolved by breakpoint cluster region (bcr) rearrangement analysis, and, if positive, would indicate Ph[1]-negative CML. CMML could be further characterized by modifying the criteria for monocytosis to include a relative value of 8% or more monocytes in the peripheral blood or bone marrow in those instances of severe leukocytosis. In CMML patients with more myelodysplasia than proliferation, i.e., a WBC count <20 × 10^9/L, an absolute monocyte count of 10^9/L or more would be required. In addition, cytochemistry, immunocytochemistry, and immunophenotyping by flow cytometry would help to differentiate CMML from RAEB. Certainly, clearer definitions and classifications will evolve when the molecular abnormalities are better understood in relation to the pathophysiological events.

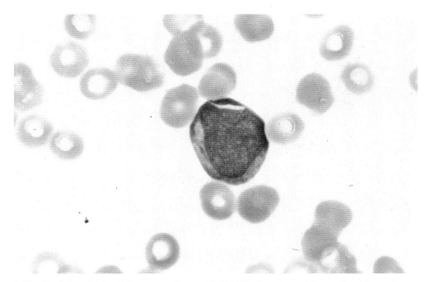

Figure 2.21   Peripheral blood from a patient with RAEB showing a blast cell with an Auer rod and multiple nucleoli. Note artifact in upper portion of nucleus. (×1,000).

Refractory Anemia with Excess Blasts in Transformation (RAEB-IT)

This subgroup (Fig. 2.21) was originally proposed because it was thought to represent early AML. However, 40% of patients do not progress to AML, but they do have a dismal median survival of only 5 months. Since patients under 50 years of age may respond well to conventional chemotherapy for AML, some hematologists recommend that RAEB-IT in patients under the age of 50 be treated as a FAB-M2.

Refractory Cytopenias Including Refractory Neutropenias (RN) and Refractory Thrombocytopenias (RT)

Although these rare disorders exist and belong within the MDSs, they have not been included in the FAB MDS classification.

In RN the neutropenia is absolute, with a count of less than 2×10^9/L. The bone marrow may be hypo-, normo-, or hypercellular, but if it is hypocellular, the cellularity must exceed 10%. Evidence of dysgranulopoiesis is present, and there is no significant increase in myeloblasts (<5% in bone marrow). Neutrophilic precursors must be present and must constitute at least 10% of marrow cells. Since isolated neutropenias in children and adults have numerous hereditary (Kostmann's syndrome, cyclic neutropenia, myelokathexis, Schwachman's syndrome, Fanconi's syndrome, etc.) and acquired causes (infections, severe sepsis, isoimmune neonatal neutropenia, drug-induced neutropenia, large granular lymphocytosis, etc.), RN becomes a diagnosis of exclusion.

In RT, the thrombocytopenia is persistent, with counts of less than 180×10^9/L. The bone marrow cellularity may be similar to that of RN. Platelets show abnormalities in size, shape, granule content, microtubule structure, and canalicu-

Table 2.2 Scoring Systems for MDS

Parameter Measured	Bournemouth Score	Worsley et al. Score	Düsseldorf Score	Goasguen et al. Score
Hemoglobin <10 g/dL	1	1	1	1
Neutrophils <2.5 × 10⁹/L or >16 × 10⁹/L*	1	1	—	—
Platelets <100 × 10⁹/L	1	1	1	1
Bone marrow blasts >5%	1	1	1	1
Lactic dehydrogenase U/L	—	—	1	—
Maximum score	4	4	4	3

*Represents the Worsley et al. modification.

lar structure. Megakaryocytes may show maturation arrest, as seen in the 5q-syndrome, with a predominance of small megakaryocytes or giant hyperseg-mented megakaryocytes. As in RN, the diagnosis is one of exclusion. A variety of hereditary (May-Hegglin anomaly, Bernard-Soulier syndrome, Wiskott-Aldrich syndrome, thrombocytopenia-absent radius syndrome) and acquited disorders (spurious thrombocytopenia, autoimmune thrombocytopenic purpura, secondary immune thrombocytopenia) and drugs must be included.

Both RN and RT may develop into a more advanced stage of MDS or acute leukemia which can then be classified by FAB criteria. Also, rare cases may present with combined neutropenia and thrombocytopenia.

SCORING SYSTEMS

Since MDS demonstrates clinical heterogeneity, a number of scoring systems and regression models have been created to predict patient outcome at presentation. Some of these scoring systems are presented in Table 2.2.

The Bournemouth score was based upon routine parameters presented in the table. Those scoring 0 or 1 (group A) had a median survival of 62 months; those scoring 2 or 3 (group B), 22 months; and those scoring 4 (group C), 4 months.

Since the majority of CMML patients have neutrophilia rather than neutropenia, Worsley et al. (1988) modified the Bournemouth scoring system by adding neutro-philia of more than 16×10^9/L. Although a granulocyte count of more than 16×10^9/L or a monocyte count of more than 2.6×10^9/L correlated with poor survival, the best prognosticator of poor survival was the modified Bournemouth (Worsley) system, as shown in Table 2.2. Those patients who scored 2 or more by the Worlsey method had a median survival of 9 months, whereas those who scored 0–1 had a survival of 32 months.

Table 2.3 Sanz et al. Scoring System for MDS

Parameter Measured	Score
Bone marrow blasts (%)	
<5	0
5–10	1
>10	2
Platelet count × 10^9/L	
<100	0
50–100	1
<50	2
Age (years)	
<60	0
>60	1
Maximum score	5

Source: Sanz GF, Sanz MA, Vallespi T, et al: Two regression models and a scoring system for predicting survival and planning treatment in myelodysplastic syndromes: A multivariate analysis of prognostic factors in 370 patients. *Blood* 74:395–408, 1989.

The only scoring system utilizing lactic dehydrogenase levels has been proposed by Aul et al. (1987) from Düsseldorf.

Goasguen et al. (1990) devised a modification of the Bournemouth score in which they eliminated consideration of the neutrophil parameters. In evaluation of 503 patients with MDS, they determined that patients with MDS who scored 0 had a median survival of 72 months, whereas those who scored 3 had a median survival of only 7 months.

Since the percentage of the bone marrow blast cells is the most important prognostic feature, Sanz et al. (1989), using a multivariate proportional hazard analysis, demonstrated that the combination of bone marrow blast percentage, hemoglobin concentration, platelet count, and age was the best predictor of survival. The Sanz et al. scoring system is shown in Table 2.3. It places greater emphasis on the bone marrow blast percentage, excludes hemoglobin and neutrophil values, but includes age as an additional parameter. The last has been criticized by some authors, since age failed to show significance by univariate or multivariate analysis in their studies. However, the Sanz et al. system has the advantage of defining more clearly patients with different percentages of blasts. Those patients with more than 5% blasts can be segregated into three risks groups with a median survival of 51 months (score of 1), 15 months (score of 2 or 3), and 4 months (score of 4 or 5). This suggests that the Sanz et al. scoring system may be more useful in the risk assessment of patients with RAEB and RAEB-IT, as well as in patients with CMML with more than 5% blasts in the bone marrow. Combining the Sanz et al. system with other prognostic factors will undoubtedly improve the clinician's ability to predict the outcome of individual patients. Additional factors that have an impact on survival include ALIP and the results of cytogenetic studies.

All of these scoring systems are relatively simple to apply, but undoubtedly newer systems or modifications of the older systems will be created as we continue to learn more about the MDSs.

BIBLIOGRAPHY

Articles

Aul C, Derigs G, Schneider W: Abstracts of the First International Symposium on Myelodysplastic Syndromes, Innsbruck, June 20–23. *Blut* 56:C1–C23, 1987.

Berndt MC, Kabral A, Grimsley P, et al: An acquired Bernard-Soulier-like platelet defect associated with juvenile myelodysplastic syndrome. *Br J Haematol* 68:97–101, 1988.

Davey FR, Erber WN, Gatter KC, et al: Abnormal neutrophils in acute myeloid leukemia and myelodysplastic syndrome. *Hum Pathol* 19:454–459, 1988.

Felman P, Bryon PA, Gentilhomme O, et al: The syndrome of abnormal chromatin clumping in leucocytes: A myelodysplastic disorder with proliferative features? *Br J Haematol* 70:49–54, 1988.

Fohlmeister I, Fischer R, Mödder B, et al: Aplastic anemia and the hypocellular myelodysplastic syndrome: Histomorphological, diagnostic, and prognostic features. *J Clin Pathol* 38:1218–1224, 1985.

Fox SB, Lorenzen J, Heryet A, et al: Megakaryocytes in myelodysplasia: An immunohistochemical study on bone marrow trephines. *Histopathology* 17:69–74, 1990.

Goasguen JE, Bennett JM, Cox C, et al: Prognostic implication and characterization of the blast cell population in the myelodysplastic syndrome. *Leuk Res* 15:1159–1165, 1991.

Goasguen JE, Garand R, Bizet M, et al: Prognostic factors of myelodysplastic syndromes: A simplified 3-D scoring system. *Leuk Res* 14:255–262, 1990.

Hast R: Sideroblasts in myelodysplasia: Their nature and clinical significance. *Scand J Haematol* 36(Suppl 45):53–55, 1986.

Hatfield SJ, Fester ED, Steytler JG: Apoptotic megakaryocyte dysplasia in the myelodysplastic syndromes. *Hematol Pathol* 6:87–93, 1992.

Imbert M, Jarry MT, Tulliez M, et al: Platelet peroxidase deficiency in a case of myelodysplastic syndrome with myelofibrosis. *J Clin Pathol* 36:1223–1228, 1983.

Islam A, Catovsky D, Goldman JM, et al: Bone marrow fiber content in acute myeloid leukaemia before and after treatment. *J Clin Pathol* 37:1259–1263, 1984.

Jaen A, Irriguible D, Milla F, et al: Abnormal chromatin clumping in leucocytes: A clue to a new subtype of myelodysplastic syndrome. *Eur J Haematol* 45:209–214, 1990.

Kawaguchi M, Nehashi Y, Aizawa S, et al: Comparative study of immunocytochemical staining versus Giemsa stain for detecting dysmegakaryopoiesis in myelodysplastic syndromes (MDS). *Eur J Haematol* 44:89–94, 1990.

Knight DK, Amos A, Layton DM, et al: Platelet associated immunoproteins in primary myelodysplastic syndromes. *Br J Haematol* (Spec Suppl):43, 1988.

Kuriyama K, Tomonaga M, Matsuo T, et al: Diagnostic significance of detecting pseudo Pelger-Huët anomalies and micromegakaryocytes in myelodysplastic syndrome. *Br J Haematol* 63:665–669, 1986.

Lambertenghi-Deliliers G, Annaloro C, Orinarri A, et al: Myelodysplastic syndromes associated with bone marrow fibrosis. *Leuk-Lymphoma* 8:51–55, 1992.

Lambertenghi-Deliliers G, Annaloro C, Oriani A, et al: Prognostic relevance of histological findings on bone marrow biopsy in myelodysplastic syndromes. *Ann Hematol* 66:85–91, 1993.

Langenhuijsen MM: Neutrophils with ring-shaped nuclei in myeloproliferative disease. *Br J Haematol* 58:227–230, 1984.

Mangi MH, Mufti GJ: Primary myelodysplastic syndromes: Diagnostic and prognostic significance of immunohistochemical assessment of bone marrow biopsies. *Blood* 79:198–205, 1992.

Mangi MH, Mufti GJ, Sahsbury JR: Abnormal localization of immature precursors (ALIP) in the bone marrow of myelodysplastic syndromes: Current state of knowledge and future directions. *Leuk Res* 15:627–639, 1991.

Mufti GJ, Figes A, Hamblin TJ, et al: Immunological abnormalities in myelodysplastic syndromes. I. Serum immunoglobulins and autoantibodies. *Br J Haematol* 63:143–147, 1986.

Muti GJ, Stevens JR, Oscier DG, et al: Myelodysplastic syndromes: A scoring system with prognostic significance. *Br J Haematol* 59:425–433, 1985.

Nand S, Godwin JE: Hypoplastic myelodysplastic syndrome. *Cancer* 62:958–964, 1988.

Rios A, Canizo MC, Sanz MA, et al: Bone marrow biopsy in myelodysplastic syndromes: Morphological characteristics and contribution to the study of prognostic factors. *Br J Haematol* 75:26–33, 1990.

Rasi V, Lintula R: Platelet function in the myelodysplastic syndromes. *Scand J Haematol* 36(Suppl 45):71–73, 1986.

Rummens JL, Verfaillie C, Criel A, et al: Elliptocytosis and schistocytosis in myelodysplasia: Report of two cases. *Acta Haematol* 75:174–177, 1986.

Ruwtu P: Granulocyte function in myelodysplastic syndromes. *Scand J Haematol* 36(Suppl 45):66–70, 1986.

Sanz GF, Sanz MA, Vallespi T, et al: Two regression models and a scoring system for predicting survival and planning treatment in myelodysplastic syndromes: A multivariate analysis of prognostic factors in 370 patients. *Blood* 74:395–408, 1989.

Thiede T, Engquist L, Billstrom R: Application of megakaryocytic morphology in diagnosing 5q-syndrome. *Eur J Haematol* 41:434–437, 1988.

Third MIC Cooperative Study Group: Recommendations for a morphologic immunologic, and cytogenetic (MIC) working classification of the primary and therapy-related myelodysplastic disorders: Report of the workshop held in Scottsdale AZ, USA, on February 23–25, 1987. *Cancer Genet Cytogenet* 32:1–10, 1988.

Tricot GJ, De Wolf-Peeters C, Hendrick B, et al: II Prognostic value of ALIP in MDS. *Br J Haematol* 58:217–225, 1984.

Tricot G, De Wolf-Peeters, Vlietinck R, et al: Bone marrow histology in myelodysplastic syndromes. II. Prognostic value of abnormal localization of immature precursors in MDS. *Br J Haematol* 58:217–225, 1984.

Tulliez M, Testa U, Rochant H, et al: Reticulocytosis, hypochromia and microcytosis: An unusual presentation of preleukemic syndrome. *Blood* 59:293–299, 1982.

Van de Weide M, Sizoo W, Krefft J, et al: Myelodysplastic syndromes: Analysis of morphological features related to the FAB-classification. *Eur J Haematol* 41:58–61, 1988.

Wong KF, Chan JK: Are dysplastic and hypogranular megakaryocytes specific markers for myelodysplastic syndrome? *Br J Haematol* 77:509–514, 1991.

Worsley A, Oscier DG, Stevens J, et al: Prognostic features of chronic myelomonocytic leukemia: A modified Bournemouth score gives the best prediction of survival. *Br J Haematol* 68:17–21, 1988.

Review Articles

Bennett JM, Catovsky D, Daniel MT, et al: Proposals for the classification of the acute leukemias. *Br J Haematol* 33:451–458, 1976.

Bennett JM, Catovsky D, Daniel MT, et al: Proposals for the classification of the myelodysplastic syndromes. *Br J Haematol* 51:189–199, 1982.

Besa EC: Myelodysplastic syndrome (refractory anemia). A perspective of the biologic, clinical and therapeutic issues. *Med Clin North Am* 76:599–617, 1992.

Cazzola M, Ponchio L, Rosti V, et al: Diagnostic approach to the myelodysplastic syndromes. *Leukemia* 6(Suppl 4):19–22, 1992.

Foucar K, Langdon RM, Armitage JO, et al: Myelodysplastic syndromes: A clinical and pathological analysis of 109 cases. *Cancer* 56:553–561, 1985.

Goasguen JE, Bennett JM: Classification and morphologic features of the myelodysplastic syndromes. *Semin Oncol* 19:4–13, 1992.

Jacobs A: Myelodysplastic syndromes: Pathogenesis, functional abnormalities, and clinical implications. *J Clin Pathol* 38:1201–1217, 1985.

Kampmeier P, Anastasi J, Vardiman JW: Issues in the pathology of the myelodysplastic syndromes. *Hematol Oncol Clin North Am* 6(3):501–522, 1992.

Kouides PA, Bennett JM: Morphology and classifications of myelodysplastic syndromes. *Hematol Oncol Clin North Am* 6(3):485–499, 1992.

Krause JR: *Bone Marrow Biopsy.* Edinburgh, Churchill Livingstone, 1981.

Noel P, Solberg LA Jr: Myelodysplastic syndromes: Pathogenesis, diagnosis and treatment. *Crit Rev Oncol Hematol* 12:193–215, 1992.

Pierre RV: *Myelodysplastic Syndromes.* Lake Louise and Banff Springs, Mayo Medical Laboratories, June 1–5, 1992.

CHAPTER **3**

Differential Diagnosis and Secondary Myelodysplastic Syndrome

BACKGROUND

Diagnosis of an MDS can, at times, be most difficult because some other diseases are also associated with bone marrow dysplasia. Most of these disorders are acquired and some are inherited. Of the acquired disorders, aplastic anemia and its sequelae resulting from immunosuppressive therapy can strongly mimic a MDS. Autoimmune or autoimmune-associated diseases, including pure red cell aplasia, chronic lymphatic leukemia, T-lymphoproliferative disorders, thyrotoxicosis, and Weber-Christian vasculitis, may ape and predispose to myelodysplasia. Drugs, including alkylating agents, and antimetabolites commonly produce dysplastic changes in the bone marrow. Various heavy metals including arsenic, lead, and zinc-induced copper deficiency may induce bizarre myelodysplastic changes. Lastly, inflammatory conditions, such as tuberculosis, and even acute leukemia may produce marrow changes mimicking MDS which at times can be extremely difficult to delineate clearly. With the resurgence of tuberculosis in this era of immunosuppression and the acquired immune deficiency syndrome (AIDS), hematologists and hematopathologists will undoubtedly see more hematological complications related to MDS.

Hereditary disorders such as Fanconi's anemia, Bloom's syndrome, ataxia-telangiectasia, Wiskott-Aldrich syndrome, and Down's syndrome, which have a propensity for hematological malignancy, but especially acute leukemia, may produce findings that mimic MDS. Also, acute nonlymphocytic leukemia has been reported in association with Kostmann's agranulocytosis, Blackfan-Diamond

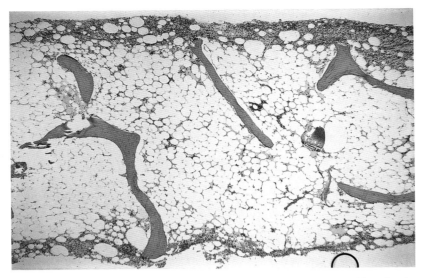

Figure 3.1 Bone marrow biopsy specimen from a patient with aplastic anemia. Note the absence of ALIP, erythroid islands, and micromegakaryocytes and megakaryoblasts. (×100)

anemia, amegakaryocytic thrombocytopenia, and Poland's syndrome. Finally, hereditary sideroblastic anemias involving the aminolevulinic acid synthetase gene on the X chromosome may produce a sideroblastic anemia mimicking RARS.

Initially the FAB group considered secondary or therapy-related MDS (t-MDS) to be identical to primary MDS. However, only one-half to one-fifth of such cases can be readily classified by the FAB criteria. One reason is that marrow blasts usually total less than 5%, and many immature dysplastic erythroid, megakaryocytic, and monocytic forms are observed. Therefore, no one cell lineage clearly predominates. In addition, the marrow may be hypocellular with increased fibrosis, resulting in a dry tap. Consequently, the bone marrow biopsy is of invaluable benefit to establish the correct diagnosis. Because of these difficulties, the Morphologic, Immunologic, and Cytogenic Cooperative Study Group (MIC) added t-MDS to the FAB classification. This new subgroup included patients with MDS associated with myelofibrosis, isolated neutropenias or thrombocytopenias, and syndromes having features of both MDS and myeloproliferative syndromes. The majority of t-MDS cases demonstrated chromosomal abnormalities involving chromosomes 5 and/or 7, either alone or in combination with other changes.

DISORDERS THAT MAY MIMIC MDS

Aplastic Anemia

Although hypocellular MDS appears to account for less than 10–15% of all cases, differentiating these cases from aplastic anemia (Fig. 3.1) can at times be extremely difficult. Most investigators consider a case of MDS hypoplastic when the bone marrow biopsy specimen exhibits cellularity of less than 25–30%. However, if the patient is more than 60 years old, some authors require the cellularity to be less than 20%. Cellularity in patients with aplastic anemia is usually less than 10%. If the FAB criteria for MDS are applied to hypocellular cases, the majority are categorized as RA and RAEB. Rare cases of RA with ringed sideroblasts or RAEB-IT have been described. Interestingly, CMML, which is characterized by a hypercellular marrow, has not been reported to have a hypocellular variant. Goasguen and Bennett (1992) have suggested the following criteria, which may be useful in diagnosing hypocellular MDS: ALIP, i.e., located centrally in the medullary tissue instead of lining the endosteal surface; an increase in immature myeloid precursors; an island of erythroblastic precursors; and the presence of micromegakaryocytes and megakaryoblasts, which may be identified by CD41 or factor VIII monoclonal antibody. Obviously, the distinction between aplastic anemia and hypocellular MDS is most important, since the correct diagnosis will dictate the clinical management and prognosis.

The difficulties in separating MDS from aplastic anemia have been addressed by Appelbaum et al. (1987), who suggested that a clonal cytogenetic abnormality in aplastic anemia is an indication that the disorder is a preleukemic syndrome. They studied 183 patients with aplastic anemia and noted that only 7 (4%) showed clonal chromosomal abnormalities frequently seen in MDS or AML, including deletion of the long arm of chromosome 5, monosomy 7, and trisomy 8. Although five patients (3%) had no cytogenetic abnormalities and subsequently developed either MDS or leukemia, they concluded that all patients with aplastic anemia may have some risk of developing leukemia. However, they further suggested that those with a cytogenetic abnormality are at especially high risk. By contrast, Moormeier et al. (1991) observed three patients with hypocellular marrow, mild dysplasia, and trisomy 6 who did not have the clinical characteristics of MDS. Also, two of the three patients responded to treatment directed at autoimmune-mediated aplastic anemia. These findings suggest that clonal cytogenetic abnormalities may not be a specific indicator of MDS. However, the finding of an abnormality common to MDS and AML, such as -5, del(5q),7,del(7q), and trisomy 8, would support a premalignant myeloid proliferation. To make matters even more difficult, some investigators have observed cases in which an aplastic bone marrow evolved to a cellular dysplastic marrow and terminated as frank acute myelogenous leukemia. These cases require careful monitoring of peripheral blood, bone marrow, cytogenetics, and molecular genetics to determine the subtle changes that underlie such an evolutionary process.

Myeloproliferative Disorder (MPD)

MDS is characterized by ineffective dysplastic hematopoiesis, usually with either normocellular or hypercellular bone marrow. By contrast, essential MPD shows effective hematopoiesis with normal or near-normal morphology in a hypercellular bone marrow and an increase in one or more peripheral blood elements. However, despite these apparently fundamental differences, some patients manifest features of both disorders in peripheral blood and bone marrow, creating great difficulty in accurately categorizing their disease. In general, such patients can be considered to fall into three groups: (1) those with MPD including chronic myelogenous leukemia (CML), in whom dysplastic, ineffective hematopoiesis occurs as a manifestation of the transformation to a more aggressive or accelerated stage; (2) those whose hematological findings straddle MPD and MDS from the onset; and (3) rarely, those who progress from a MDS to a chronic MPD. Those patients who cannot be classified into one of the five FAB groups should be designated as having unclassified MDS. Also, if a myeloproliferative element exists, it should be recognized and documented.

When CML transforms into an accelerated or blast phase, hematopoiesis becomes dysplastic in many patients and anemia, thrombocytopenia, and, rarely, leukopenia ensue. Transformation of CML associated with dysplasia is easily recognized when a history of a chronic phase exists, but occasional patients have a silent or unrecognized chronic period with initial presentation of transformation. In these latter patients distinction of MPD from MDS may be difficult, and the diagnosis will depend on the demonstration of the Ph[1] and/or *BCR/ABL* rearrangement.

The classical prototype for patients with features that straddle MDS and chronic MPD is CMML, which was discussed in some detail in Chapter 2. CMML was placed in the MDS category by the FAB group primarily because of the striking dysplasia, and also because cytopenias of one or more peripheral blood elements are not uncommon. Also, the clinical course, the rate and pattern of leukemic transformation, and the high incidence of point mutations in the *RAS* oncogene family support a myelodysplastic process. Nevertheless, this position is not accepted by all investigators, since myeloproliferative features predominate in a substantial number of patients. Recently, Wessels et al. (1993) have reported two patients with t(5;12)(q31;p12) who were Ph[1] negative and *BCR/ABL* rearrangement negative, with clinical and morphological features of both CML and CMML. Since three previous cases with that translocation had been reported, the authors suggested that t(5;12)(q31p12) may typify a distinct subgroup of myeloid disorders. Wiedeman et al. (1988) proposed the term *atypical chronic myelogenous leukemia* for these disorders defined as a leukemic disorder with dysplastic granulocytes; absent or few basophils; a proportion of promyelocytes, myelocytes, and metamyelocytes exceeding 10%; and, often, monocytosis and thrombocytopenia. Although acceptance of the term *atypical chronic myelogenous leukemia* or *atypical granulocytic leukemia* is growing for this heterogeneous group of disorders, additional large series of such patients need to be collected and carefully analyzed.

In addition to those cases that progress from chronic MPD to a dysplastic, more aggressive, transformed state and those that share features of both chronic MPD and MDS, Ohyashiki et al. (1993) have described two patients with MDS who progressed to chronic MPD. Both patients had anemia and mild neutropenia without thrombocytopenia at the time of diagnosis of MDS. However, after prolonged treatment with vitamin D$_3$, they developed a leukothrombocytosis that mimicked chronic MPD and responded to hydroxyurea. The authors suggest that these patients, along with similar patients, may constitute a category distinct from typical MDS and chronic MDS. However, additional cases need to be studied and the effect of treatment on producing such a disorder determined before such a category is created.

MDS versus AML and Erythroleukemia

Frequently, the distinction between MDS and AML may be very difficult. De novo AML with trilineage myelodysplastic features may represent either progression of clinically occult MDS or simultaneous occurrence. Since some early AMLs may have blast percentages and morphology similar to those of chronic MDS, they are usually diagnosed as having RAEB-IT. The response of AML with associated MDS changes to treatment is controversial. Some studies found fewer reduction remissions, but a recent study did not demonstrate that dysplastic changes in AML affected the outcome.

Finally, most recent studies by Morris et al. (1992) have identified an AML with increased megakaryocytes and severe trilineage dysplasia with karyotypic findings of t(3;5)(q25.1;q34). Although the chromosome 5 breakpoint of the t(3;5) was considerably telomeric to the CSFIR/PDGFRB locus, the authors suggested that future efforts to identify the genes affected by the t(3;5) should focus on the 5q segment.

Another area of great diagnostic difficulty is FAB M6, since the criteria include only those cases in which erythroid precursors account for more than 50% of the marrow cells and myeloblasts account for more than 30% of the nonerythroid elements. These criteria eliminate pure erythroleukemia and mixed (myeloblastic and proerythroblastic) erythroleukemia, relegating them to the MDS category. Recent studies by Kowal-Vern et al. (1992) have shown that patients with a predominance of proerythroblasts have a much poorer prognosis than those with a predominance of myeloblasts. They propose that the erythroleukemia with myeloblastic predominance be designated FAB M6a and those with the proerythroblastic predominance called FAB M6b. Evidently, morphology correlates with cytogenetics and survival, since patients with more than two karyotypic abnormalities showed a higher percentage of proerythroblasts (FAB M6b) and poor survival, whereas those with fewer proerythroblasts and myeloblastic predominance (FAB M6a) revealed only one or two karyotypic abnormalities and a longer survival time (Fig. 3.2). Therefore, cytogenetic analysis seems especially imperative in those difficult cases of AML with trilineage dysplasia and those of FAB M6.

MISCELLANEOUS PROBLEMS IN DIAGNOSIS

MDS of Childhood

Children with MDS show pancytopenia, although hepatosplenomegaly and granulocytic sarcoma are far more common than in the adult population. Even though all MDS types with the exception of RARS have been reported, predominance of the aggressive types is high. Mean survival is usually less than 1 year, and the majority of patients show a Bournemouth score of 3 to 4. Cytogenetic analyses in some patients have revealed karyotypic abnormalities involving chromosomes 7, 8, and 17. Because of the aggressive nature of this disorder in children and the poor response to intensive chemotherapy, early bone marrow transplantation seems to be indicated (Fig. 3.3).

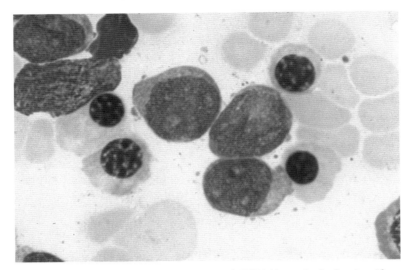

Figure 3.2a   A bone marrow aspirate from a patient with FAB M6a erythroleukemia with myeloblasts surrounded by nucleated red blood cells. Note the granules in the myeloblast in the upper left center. (×1,000).

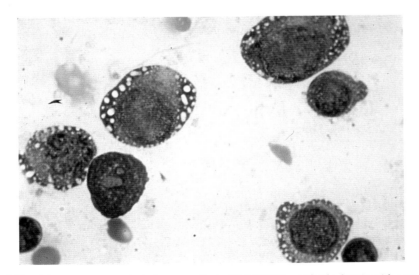

Figure 3.2b   A bone marrow aspirate from a patient with FAB M6b erythroleukemia with a predominance of proerythroblasts. Note the round nuclei with sharp nuclear membrane, vacuolated deep basophilic cytoplasm, and lack of granules. This is usually classified as an MDS, since erythroid elements are excluded from the current FAB criteria for M6. (×1,000).

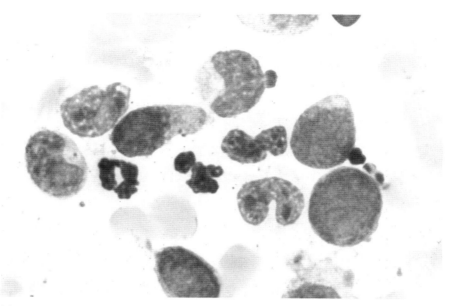

Figure 3.3 Bone marrow aspirate from a child with CMML. Note the blasts, monocytes, agranular bands and neutrophil. (×1,000).

Human Immunodeficiency Virus (HIV)-Related MDS

Myelodysplastic changes are being increasingly described in the literature in patients with AIDS. Karcher and Frost (1991) reported on 216 bone marrows in 178 HIV-infected patients. The most common findings were hypercellularity (53%) and dysplasia involving at least one cell line (69%), with erythrocytic, megakaryocytic, and dysgranulocytic dysplasia in 56%, 31%, and 18% of specimens, respectively. Dyserythropoietic features included nuclear irregularity, multinucleation, and intranuclear chromatin bridging. Megakaryocytic dysplasia included dwarf forms, nuclear hyposegmentation, and nuclear fragmentation. However, a study by Thiele et al. (1992), who evaluated AIDS patients without prior myelotoxic therapy by morphometric and immunohistochemical analysis, failed to reveal myelodysplastic changes in the megakaryocytic lineage. They did not observe a predominance of micromegakaryocytes and showed a conspicuous absence of promegakaryocytes. Others have demonstrated apoptosis in AIDS and chronic MPD patients manifested by compact, denuded megakaryocyte nuclei surrounded by a thin rim of cytoplasm. Granulocytic series showed nuclear-cytoplasmic asynchrony, and occasional marrow aspirates exhibited hypogranular or multinucleated maturing cells.

The mechanisms involved in HIV-related myelodysplasia are not clear. Multiple factors including drug toxicity, opportunistic infections, and HIV itself have been suggested as causative factors. Although the morphological features in some AIDS patients may resemble those of primary MDS; one major difference is that progression to acute leukemia is highly unlikely. Additional cases of AIDS need to be evaluated (excluding those subdued by myelotoxic therapy) to determine

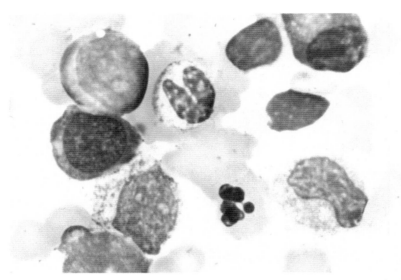

Figure 3.4 Bone marrow aspirate from an AIDS patient demonstrating an agranular band and marked nuclear dyskinesis in an erythroid precursor (lower center). (×1,000).

the exact effect of the HIV and/or opportunistic infections on the bone marrow elements. Clearly, multifactorial mechanisms are in operation in the hematological findings so far reported in AIDS (Fig. 3.4).

Extramedullary Disease and Transformation

Extramedullary blast transformation in MDS occurs most frequently in the skin, but transformation at other sites, including lymph nodes, spleen, liver, colon, nasal sinuses, breast, and brain, has been reported. Although extramedullary manifestations of MDS are well known in CMML, granulocytic sarcoma has also been reported in RAEB and RAEB-IT. The diagnosis of such lesions depends upon biopsy and identification of immature myeloid cells by means of either cytochemical stains or immunological markers. Chloroacetate esterase (Leder's stain) may present problems in that blast cells frequently do not stain. Therefore, myeloperoxidase on touch preparations and/or tissue anti-immunomyeloperoxidase should be used. Neimann et al. (1981) used antilysoenzyme immunoperoxidase stains and found them particularly useful in granulocytic sarcoma. Other cutaneous lesions such as Sweet's syndrome and cutaneous vasculitis may occur in MDS and mimic granulocytic sarcoma. Although granulocytic sarcoma developing in MDS is uncommon, it is not rare; 4.3% of MDS patients in one series developed this complication. This is comparable to the incidence reported in chronic granulocytic leukemia. Granulocytic sarcoma in MDS has an ominous prognostic significance; more than 50% of cases progress to AML within a few months, and median survival is only 2.5 months. Therefore, most clinicians believe that granulocytic sarcoma in MDS warrants immediate treatment for AML. Although identification of clonal cytogenetic abnormalities in MDS portends a higher risk of disease progression, cytogenetic analysis of MDS with granulocytic sarcoma

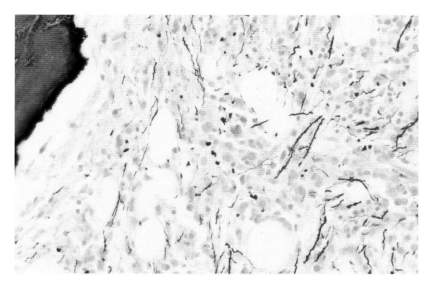

Figure 3.5   Reticulin stain of a bone marrow biopsy specimen demonstrates increased reticulin fibers in a patient with treatment-induced RAEB. This represents early mild fibrosis. (×400).

disclosed a normal karyotype in one series. Therefore, a diagnosis of granulocytic sarcoma in MDS becomes an important marker for disease acceleration. Why soft tissue or extramedullary sites should represent the initial site of disease progression in some cases of MDS is unknown.

MDS with Myelofibrosis

Myelofibrosis refers to the finding of a focal or generalized increase in the number and thickness of reticulin fibers observed in bone marrow biopsy specimens by silver impregnation stain. This represents precollagen, whereas fibers staining blue by trichrome stain represent more advanced true collagen. Some hematopathologists grade fibrosis from 1 or 2+ (mild to moderate) to 4+ (trichrome collagen positive), with the majority of patients with MDS and fibrosis being either 3+ (trichrome collagen negative) or 4+. Mild to moderate myelofibrosis occurs in up to 50% of patients with MDS, whereas severe myelofibrosis is seen in only 11–15%. Although myelofibrosis occurs in all five primary FAB subclassifications of MDS, its incidence is much greater in t-MDS (Fig. 3.5). Mild and marked fibrosis have been reported to occur in up to 85% and 50% of t-MDS, respectively.

Patients with MDS and myelofibrosis have pancytopenia, minimal organomegaly, and a hypercellular bone marrow with marked fibrosis, trilineage dysplasia, and atypical megakaryocytic proliferation with a predominance of small forms that have hypolobated nuclei. Recently, Lambertenghi et al. (1992) evaluated 106 MDS patients and characterized three patterns of bone marrow blastic infiltration as "diffuse," "cluster," and "large." Nineteen of the 106 patients who demonstrated extensive bone marrow fibrosis were characterized by cluster blastic infiltration and megakaryocytic hyperplasia. Leukemic transformation did not occur in any of the cluster cases with severe myelofibrosis, but it did occur in the large cases predominantly diagnosed as RAEB-IT. However, survival was equally poor in these two groups because of early leukemic transformation (large cases) and bone marrow failure (fibrosis cluster cases). The FAB classification did not significantly correlate with the prognosis in these two groups. Furthermore, the authors stated that patients with cluster bone marrow infiltration represented a separate MDS subset characterized by unique clinicopathological and prognostic features. Since many of these patients are elderly, conroversy as to the best therapeutic approach exists. In contrast to these primary MDSs with severe fibrosis, secondary MDSs with full-blown fibrosis seem to represent a variety of preleukemic conditions and do not form a clear-cut clinicopathological entity.

Besides the above difficulties in accurately assessing bone marrow fibrosis in MDS, other diagnostic entities including primary myelofibrosis with myeloid metaplasia (MMM) or myelosclerosis with myeloid metaplasia; an accelerated phase of CML; postpolycythemic myeloid metaplasia; AML, especially acute megakaryoblastic leukemia (FAB M7); and AML with trilineage dysplasia and the rare entity of acute myelofibrosis have created difficult diagnostic conundrums.

MMM can be distinguished from MDS with fibrosis by the presence of prominent splenomegaly, extramedullary hematopoiesis, and lack of myelodysplastic features. Malignant myelosclerosis (also known as *acute myelosclerosis*) may be the most difficult differential diagnostic problem. Myelosclerosis is a condition characterized by obliteration of the normal bone marrow cavity by the formation of small spicules of bone. It is characterized by minimal to absent splenomegaly, pancytopenia with minimal anisopoikilocytosis, and rapid progression to death. The bone marrow findings demonstrate panmyelosis with a predominance of megakaryocytes, immaturity of all three cell lines, and marked myelofibrosis. Controversy exists as to whether myelosclerosis does in fact represent a single entity. Some authors contend that it represents a heterogeneous group of diseases, including FAB M7 AML, an accelerated phase of primary myelofibrosis, or MDS with myelofibrosis. The accelerated phase of CML may be separated on the basis of the history, existing splenomegaly, and the presence of Ph[1] and/or *BCR/ABL* rearrangement.

Acute leukemia, especially FAB M7 and AML with trilineage dysplasia, must be separated from acute myelosclerosis and MDS with myelofibrosis. Since bone marrow aspirate material may not be available, peripheral blood and a well-prepared biopsy specimen are invaluable for the disgnosis. If 30% or more of the cells in the peripheral blood and/or bone marrow aspirate are blasts, the diagnosis is AML. The use of flow cytometry, cytochemical and immunohistochemical stains, and electron microscopy for platelet peroxidase will help delineate the type of acute leukemia. The antibodies utilized should include those for factor VIII–related antigens, platelet glycoproteins IIB/IIIA (CD 41), platelet GP IX (CD42a), and GP 1b (CD 42b).

Myelofibrosis seems to represent either a nonspecific or a reactive response to a variety of bone marrow injuries and/or stimuli. This conclusion is supported by the fact that bone marrow fibroblasts cultured from patients with chronic MPD demonstrate different karyotypes and heterogeneous G6PD isoenzyme electrophoretic patterns. Apparently, the pathogenesis of increased fibrosis in hematopoietic disorders has been attributed to platelet-derived growth factors and platelet-transforming growth factor β, which stimulate fibroblastic proliferation, as well as platelet factor IV, which inhibits collagen breakdown. This hypothesis is supported by the association between atypical megakaryocytic proliferations and marked myelofibrosis. The quintessential disease demonstrating such findings is acute megakaryocytic leukemia (FAB M7).

Lymphoproliferative Disease

Lymphoid infiltrates may be observed in biopsy specimens from MDS patients. Usually they are composed of small, mature lymphocytes without cytologic atypia and do not have a paratrabecular distribution. Therefore, a diagnosis of a concurrent lymphoproliferative disorder in a patient with MDS must be made with caution. However, Copplestone et al. (1986) assembled a series of 20 patients who had MDS at the time of diagnosis of their lymphoid or plasma cell neoplasm. These included a wide range of B- and T-cell neoplasms that involved all five FAB MDS classes. The lymphoplasmacytic disorders comprised chronic lymphocytic leukemia; centroblastic/centrocytic, T-pleomorphic, and lymphoplasmacytic malignant lymphoma; multiple myeloma, and smoldering myeloma. Although Stark et al. (1987) challenged the coexistence of MDS and lymphoproliferative disease, Hamblin constructed a working hypothesis proposing that MDS could arise from an initial event which selects a clone of stem cells that retains the capacity to differentiate into mature lymphoid and myeloid cells. This clone has a growth advantage over other clones but carries genetic defects that accumulate and progress. Each genetic event makes subsequent events more likely, so that culmination in frank malignancy is always a distinct possibility (Fig. 3.6). The authors suggest that disorders such as benign monoclonal gammopathy and stage A0 in chronic lymphocytic leukemia may represent the lymphoid equivalent of RA in the myeloid line.

Besides coexistent lymphoproliferative disorders, large granular lymphocytosis (T-gamma lymphoproliferative disorders) may sometimes produce myelodysplastic changes within the peripheral blood and bone marrow that mimic MDS. It is most important to make this diagnosis, if present, since such patients may respond to steroids (Fig. 3.7).

5q- Syndrome

In 1974, Van den Berghe and associates described three patients with a deletion of the long arm of chromosome 5 (5q-). This 5q syndrome was characterized by refractory anemia with macrocytic red blood cells, low or low normal WBC counts, normal or elevated platelet counts, and hypolobated micromegakaryocytic hyperplasia (Fig. 3.8). The median age at diagnosis is usually over 65 years, with a clear female predominance. Large numbers of patients are transfusion dependent, but significant neutropenia or thrombocytopenia is rare. By the FAB classification, the majority of cases fall into the RA category. However, the 5q- syndrome is distributed across all subtypes of MDS and is found in AML. It seems to be particularly frequent in therapy-related cases. Apparently, not all patients with 5q- syndrome have a distinct syndrome, nor do all enjoy prolonged survival. Matthew et al. (1993) noted that the incidence of transformation to acute leukemia (which was uniformly fatal) was 16% in 43 consecutive patients. They observed that neither survival nor the risk of leukemic transformation was predictable from initial

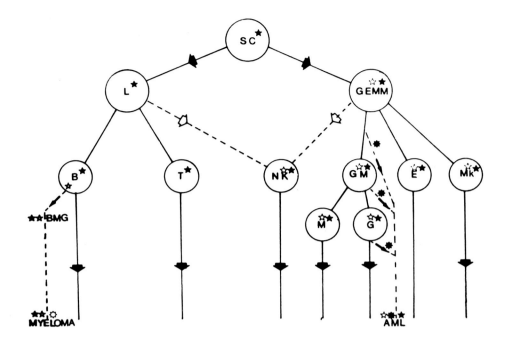

Figure 3.6   Schematic diagram of hematopoiesis representing the acquisition of successive genetic errors (starred) in the development of acute leukemia and myeloma on a myelodysplastic background. SC = stem cell; L = lymphoblast; B = B lymphocyte; T = T lymphocyte; GEMM = multipotent progenitor cell; NK = natural killer cell; GM = colony-forming unit granulocyte/macrophage; E = erythroblast; MK = megakaryoblast; G = myeloblast; M = monoblast; AML = acute myeloid leukemia. (From Hamblin TJ: Immunological abnormalities in the myelodysplastic syndromes. In Schmalzl F, Mufti GJ [eds]: *Myelodysplastic Syndromes*. Berlin, Springer-Verlag, 1992, pp 25–30. Reprinted with permission.)

clinical parameters, including FAB classification, Bournemouth score, and degree of aneuploidy. Nevertheless, if large groups are studied, many patients with the features described by Van den Berghe et al. are observed. Although the genes mapped to 5q 31 may function as leukemic suppressor genes and include the genes encoding CSF-2, 1L-3, 1L-4, 1L-5, and 1L-9; to date mutations of these genes in leukemic cells have not been identified. Since the clinical features of myeloid diseases associated with del(5q) are variable (MDS versus leukemia), once the involved gene is identified, it will be important to determine whether the same gene is involved in both types of myeloid disorders. Treatment of patients with the 5q- syndrome with corticosteroids, androgens, cis-retinoic acid, pyridoxine, and danazol has been largely unsuccessful.

SECONDARY MDS OR t-MDS

Approximately 10% of all patients with MDS have previously been subjected to potentially mutagenic therapy, usually in the form of alkylating agents or radia-

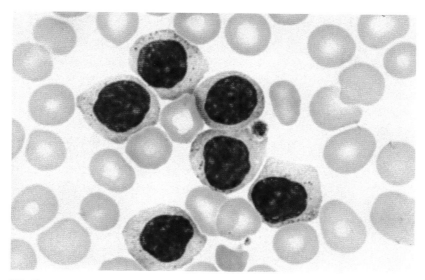

Figure 3.7   Bone marrow aspirate from a patient with large granular lymphocytosis. Note the large granular lymphocytes. Patients with this disorder may have myelodysplastic changes mimicking MDS. Therefore, it is most important to examine both peripheral blood and bone marrow aspirates for these cells in cases of MDS (×1,000).

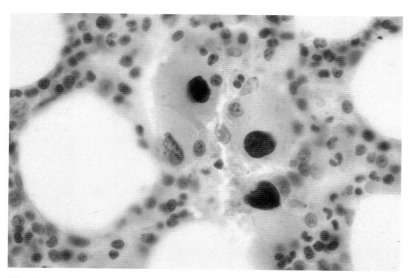

Figure 3.8   Bone marrow biopsy specimen from a patient with the 5q- syndrome. Note the numerous small, single, nucleated megakaryocytes (×400).

tion. Initially, the FAB classification regarded t-MDS as indistinguishable from primary MDS. However, only one-fifth to one-half of these cases can be easily classified by FAB criteria. The reasons are that no single dysplastic cell line predominates; the bone marrow is hypocellular with fibrosis; and dry taps predominate, usually producing insufficient aspirate material for qualitative analysis. The interval between initiation of such therapy and the onset of t-MDS ranges from 12 to 102 months (median, 53 months), and the interval between diagnosis of MDS and onset of AML ranges from 3 to 20 months (median, 7 months). Survival following diagnosis of t-MDS is dismal, with a range of only 4 to 11 months.

Recently, therapy-related AML and t-MDS in patients treated with epipodophyllotoxins over a 6-year cumulative period have been reported to be within the range previously reported for alkylator-based regimens. Since epipodophyllotoxins have an important role in the treatment of several types of adult and pediatric tumors, the National Cancer Institute has developed a monitoring plan to obtain reliable estimates of the risk of t-AML/MDS. Other drugs involved less frequently in t-AML/MDS include procarbazine, azathioprine, and nitrosoureas.

Environmental or occupational exposure to benzene or benzene-based compounds has been found to be a risk factor for the development of MDS or acute leukemia. Epidemiological data on more than 3,500 shoe and rubber industry workers showed that the risk of developing MDS or acute leukemia in this group is 5 to 20 times greater than that of the general population. Aksay (1985) has reported on 53 patients who developed MDS or acute leukemia after exposure to benzene. The average duration of exposure was 10.2 years (range, 4 months to 25 years) before cytopenias developed. The time to leukemic transformation after that period varied from 6 months to 6 years. In vitro, benzene can cause cytogenetic damage in small concentrations. The current legislated safe limit for benzene, which was 10 ppm, has been changed to 1 ppm. Exposure to ethylene oxide and petroleum products has also been associated with a higher incidence of MDS and acute leukemia.

Major studies on t-AML/MDS have suggested that three stages of evolution exist: myelodysplastic pancytopenia with less than 5% myeloblasts in the bone marrow, frank MDS resembling RAEB or RAEB-IT, and overt AML.

Chromosomal abnormalities occur in 64–85% of patients with t-MDS. Loss of chromosomal material is the most frequently encountered abnormality, usually involving chromosomes 5 and 7 (-5,-7). By contrast, the chromosome most frequently added is 8 (+8). In many cases, these abnormalities are complexed with other numeric or structural defects. Specific abnormalities or groupings often correlate with prior specific therapy (-5,-7,7q -) with chemotherapy alone or with radiation therapy; 5q- and other chromosomal defects with radiotherapy alone; and translocation and deletions in chromosome 11 at band q23 with epipodophyllotoxins, notably etoposide (VP-16) or teniposide (VM-26).

BIBLIOGRAPHY

Articles

Aksay M: Benzene as a leukemogenic and carcinogenic agent. *Am J Ind Med* 8:9–20, 1985.

Appelbaum FR, Barrall J, Storb R, et al: Clonal cytogenetic abnormalities in patients with otherwise typical aplastic anemia. *Exp Hematol* 15:1134–1139, 1987.

Ballen K, Gilliland DG, Shulman LN: Dysplastic bone marrow morphology in acute myeloblastic leukemia does not predict prognosis or correlate with history of myelodysplasia. *Blood* 78(Suppl):46a, 1991.

Bennett JM, Catovsky D, Daniel MT, et al: Proposals for the classification of the myelodysplastic syndromes. *Br J Haematol* 51:189–199, 1982.

Bennett JM, Moloney WC, Greene MH, et al: Acute myeloid leukemia and other myelopathic disorders following treatment with alkylating agents. *Hematol Pathol* 1:99–104, 1987.

Brito-Babapulle F, Catovsky D, Galton DA: Clinical and laboratory features of *de novo* acute myeloid leukemia with trilineage myelodysplasia. *Br J Haematol* 66:445–450, 1987.

Brodeur GM: The *NF-1* gene in myelopoiesis and childhood myelodysplastic syndrome. *N Engl J Med* 330:637–639, 1994.

Copplestone JA, Mufti GJ, Hamblin TJ, et al: Immunological abnormalities in myelodysplastic syndromes. II. Co-existent lymphoid or plasma cell neoplasms: A report of 20 cases unrelated to chemotherapy. *Br J Haematol* 63:149–159, 1986.

Cuneo A, Van Orshoven A, Michaux JL, et al: Morphologic, immunologic, and cytogenetic studies in erythroleukemia: Evidence for multilineage involvement and identification of two distinct cytogenetic-clinicopathological types. *Br J Haematol* 75:346–354, 1990.

De Planque MM, Kluin-Nelemens HC, Van Krieken HJ, et al: Evolution of acquired severe aplastic anaemia to myelodysplasia and subsequent leukaemia in adults. *Br J Haematol* 70:55–62, 1988.

Dolan G, Reid MM: Congenital sideroblastic anemia in two girls. *J Clin Pathol* 44:464–465, 1991.

Goasguen JE, Bennett JM: Classification and morphologic features of the myelodysplastic syndromes. *Semin Oncol* 19:4–13, 1992.

Hamblin TJ, Copplestone JA, Mufti GJ, et al: Coexistent lymphoid or plasma cell neoplasms. *Br J Haematol* 65:367–377, 1987.

Hatfill SJ, Fester ED, Steyler JG: Apoptotic megakaryocyte dysplasia in the myelodysplastic syndrome. *Hematol Pathol* 6:87–93, 1992.

Hicsönmez G, Özsoylu S: Poland's syndrome and leukemia (letter). *Am J Dis Child* 136:1098–1099, 1982.

Hirsch-Ginsberg C, LeMaistre AC, Kantarjian H, et al: RAS mutations are rare events in Philadelphia chromosome-negative/*bcr* gene rearrangement-negative chronic myelogenous leukemia, but are prevalent in chronic myelomonocytic leukemias. *Blood* 76:1214–1219, 1990.

Hogstedt C, Aringer L, Gustavsson A: Epidemiologic support for ethylene oxide as a cancer causing agent. *JAMA* 255:1575–1578, 1986.

Juneja SK, Imbert M, Jouault H, et al: Haematological features of primary myelodysplastic syndromes (PMDS) at initial presentation: A study of 118 cases. *J Clin Pathol* 36:1129–1135, 1983.

Karcher DS, Frost AR: The bone marrow in human immunodeficiency virus (HIV)-related disease. Morphology and clinical correlation. *Am J Clin Pathol* 95:63–71, 1991.

CD33, and peroxidase. Common lymphoid monoclonal antibodies include CD19, CD10, and Tdt. The latter may also be expressed in paraffin-embedded tissue. Interestingly, Tdt expression is increased in some bone marrow of MDS patients. This needs to be further investigated but probably reflects the pluripotential origin of this disorder. Guyotat et al. (1990) studied CD34, an early stem cell/myeloid differentiation marker, in MDS and found it positive in only the RAEB subtype. Its presence was associated with progression to leukemia and shorter survival, similar to the prognostic implication in AML.

Immunological techniques have also been applied to characterize megakaryocytes since they may resemble lymphoid cells morphologically. These cells can easily be identified on air-dried smears with antibodies prepared against platelet-specific glycoprotein (gp) IIb/IIIa (CD41), gp IX (CD42a), gp Ib (CD42b), or gp IIIa (CD61). Also, immunohistochemical reaction can be used to detect factor VIII.

Erythroid progenitors can be identified by monoclonal antibodies to glycophorin A, the transferrin receptor (CD71), HLe (CD45), and hemoglobin A.

The cytochemical stains that may be employed to assist in diagnosing the MDSs include the following (Table 4.1):

1. Iron stain
2. Silver stain
3. Periodic acid–Schiff (PAS)
4. Reticulin stain
5. Masson's trichrome stain
6. Myeloperoxidase (MPEX)
7. Chloroacetate esterase (CAE)
8. Alpha naphthyl butyrate esterase (B-EST)
9. Alpha naphthyl acetate esterase (A-EST)
10. Combined esterase (C-EST)
11. Leukocyte alkaline phosphatase (LAP)

In addition, various monoclonal and polyclonal antibodies have been used against various cluster designations, cell markers, and enzymes in the more difficult cases of MDSs. These include:

1. Myeloid: CD15, CD13, CD14, CD33, MPEX
2. Lymphoid: CD19, CD10
3. Stem cell: CD34
4. Megakaryocytic: CD41, CD42a, CD42b, CD61, factor VIII
5. Erythroid: CD45, CD71, glycophorin A, hemoglobin A
6. Terminal deoxynucleotidyl transferase (Tdt)

IRON STAIN

Iron stain is based on the Prussian blue reaction. Ionic iron reacts with acid ferrocynanide to give a blue color. The cells are usually counterstained with

Table 4.1   Cell Specificity and Clinical Application of Cytochemical and/or Histochemical Reactions in the MDSs

Cytochemical and/or Histochemical Reaction	Cell Specificity	Clinical Application
Iron stain	Erythroid series (ringed sideroblast) Histiocytes	MDS especially RARS, M6
Silver stain	Erythroid series (ringed sideroblasts) Nuclear organizer region	Iron-deficient MDS, M6
Periodic acid–Schiff (PAS)	Erythroid series	MDS, M6, ALL
Reticulin stain	Precollagen	MDS, MPD, CML, Hairy cell leukemia, mast cell disease
Masson's trichrome stain	Collagen	MDS, MPD, CML, hairy cell leukemia, mast cell disease
Myeloperoxidase	Granulocytes, monocytes	MDS, AML, blast crisis CML
Chloracetate esterase (CAE)	Granulocytes	MDS, MPD, granulocytic sarcoma
Alpha-naphthyl butyrate esterase (B-EST)	Monocytes, histiocytes, helper T cells	CMML, M4, M5, T-lymphoid malignancies
Alpha-naphthyl acetate esterase (A-EST) + NaF	Monocytes, histiocytes, megakaryocytes, helper T cells	CMML, M4, M5, M7 with B-EST, T-lymphoid malignancies
Combined esterase (C-EST)	Granulocytic, monocytic, histiocytic	CMML, sideroblastosis in MDS
Leukocyte alkaline phosphatase (LAP)	Neutrophils, osteoblasts, mantle zone B lymphocytes	CML, CNL, MPD, MDS, mantle zone lymphoma
Terminal deoxynucleotidyl transferase (Tdt)	Lymphoblasts, some myeloblasts	MDS, ALL, AML, CML blast crisis, T-lymphoblastic lymphoma

nuclear fast red or basic fuchsin. Bone marrow aspirates are routinely stained to evaluate the presence of both normal and abnormal iron. The stain identifies abnormal ringed sideroblasts that occur in the MDSs and erythroleukemias. The pathological ferric iron is located in the mitochondria of the erythroblast and rings the nucleus in a necklace like pattern. At least five blue granules that circumscribe at least two-thirds of the circumference of the nucleus are needed before the erythroblast is classified as a ringed sideroblast. (Controversy exists concerning these criteria; see Chapter 2.) Greater than 15% of all nucleated erythrocytes must be ringed sideroblasts in all cases of RARS. Seo et al. (1993), in evaluating a large series of patients with MDSs, revealed that 100% of cases of RARS, 46% of RA, 62% of RAEB, 65% of RAEB-IT, 57% of CMML, 73% of secondary MDS, and 36% of non-MDS hematological disorders showed some ringed sideroblasts. Besides RARS, 15% of RAEB-IT, 14% of CMML, and 27% of secondary MDS cases demonstrated more than 15% ringed sideroblasts. Ringed sideroblasts and pathological sideroblasts are depicted in Fig. 4.1.

SILVER STAIN

Ringed sideroblasts may still be demonstrable by silver stains in cases of sideroblastic anemia with associated iron deficiency anemia. Since the iron in the mitochondria is in the form of ferric phosphate, it is possible that the silver stain demonstrates the phosphate moiety and not the iron. Besides this staining feature, silver may also detect the presence of calcium, melanin, argyrophilic proteins associated with the nucleolar organizer region, and possibly other substances that will reduce silver salts. Nevertheless, misidentification of ringed sideroblasts is unlikely, provided that the cells under study are identified as nucleated red cell precursors.

Although the precise chemical basis for silver staining of ringed sideroblasts is not known, increased amounts of phosphates are apparently present in the abnormal mitochondria of MDS patients with low iron stores. This is supported by the work of Grasso et al. (1980), who showed by energy-dispersive x-ray analysis that mitochondria of ringed sideroblasts contain both iron and phosphorus. They postulated that the iron is present as ferric phosphate. Ringed sideroblasts demonstrated by silver staining are shown in Fig. 4.2.

PERIODIC ACID–SCHIFF (PAS)

The PAS reaction is widely used to identify intracellular and cytoplasmic carbohydrates, including glycogen, mucopolysaccharides, mucoproteins, glycoproteins, and glycolipids.

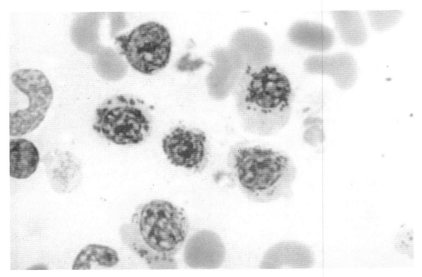

Figure 4.1a Note the numerous classical ringed sideroblasts in the bone marrow aspirate of a patient with acute erythroleukemia (Di Guglielmo's disease, M6b) (×1,000).

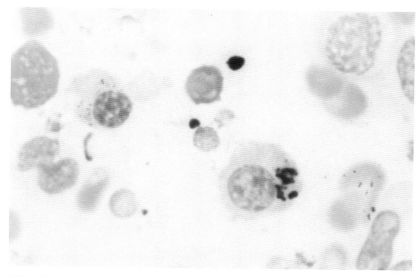

Figure 4.1b   Note the pathological sideroblast in the bone marrow aspirate of a patient with RARS. The large granular iron deposits show a polar concentration. Some hematologists and hematopathologists include these in the count of ringed sideroblasts (×1,000).

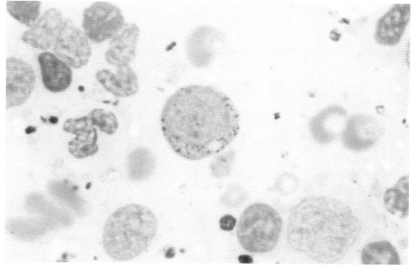

Figure 4.1c   Note the large, immature cell (most likely a proerythroblast) with iron granules surrounding the nucleus in a patient with RARS. It is most unusual to see erythroid precursors this immature containing iron or demonstrating a ringed contour BM (×1,000).

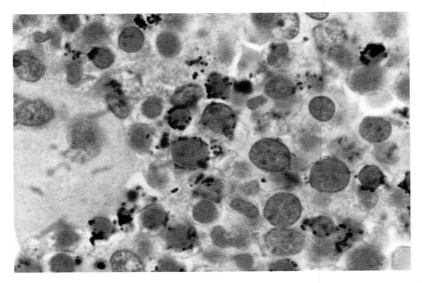

Figure 4.2 Numerous ringed sideroblasts shown by silver staining in a patient with an MDS. It is postulated that the silver stains the phosphate moiety in patients who are iron deficient and have ringed sideroblasts. BM (×1,500). (Courtesy of Kyi T. Tham.)

In the biochemical reaction, periodic acid oxidizes the 1-2 glycol grouping or its amino or alkylamino groups by clearing C—C bonds to produce aldehyde and an oxidation product. The Schiff reagent reacts with the oxidation product that is not diffusible and is present in sufficient concentration to result in a colored substitute dye. Basic fuchsin is often used and gives a magenta color, although the color may vary from pink to red to magenta.

PAS-positive erythroblasts are often seen in cases of primary and secondary MDS, the only exception being cases of CMML. However, PAS-positive erythroblasts are usually found in only small numbers (<5%). The staining pattern in erythroblasts in MDS may be similar to that observed in erythroleukemia; the PAS-positive material is coarse and granular (block) in proerythroblasts, and fine and diffuse (blush) in cells of later stages. Although PAS positivity in erythroblasts may occur in benign conditions such as iron deficiency anemia, thalassemia, and chronic renal failure, the PAS-positive material disappears after successful treatment. PAS combined with the iron stain and C-EST in evaluating cases of MDS may be very helpful. A PAS reaction on the bone marrow is shown in Fig. 4.3.

RETICULIN STAIN

Gomori's silver impregnation, a histochemical reaction, is used to evaluate precollagen-type fibrosis in the bone marrow biopsy specimen. The bone marrow biopsy specimen in MDS frequently reveals a slight alteration in the reticulin stroma which has no clinical significance. However, in a minority of cases, a full-blown bone marrow fibrosis may be observed. Primary MDS patients with extensive

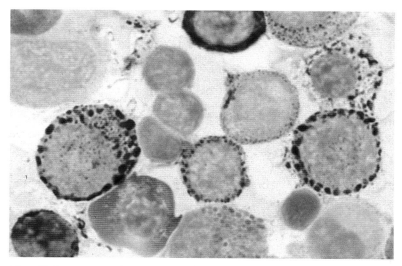

Figure 4.3a PAS reaction on bone marrow from a patient with acute erythroleukemia (M6b) (Di Guglielmo's disease). Note the grnaular and block positivity in the large proerythroblasts and the blush positivity in a more mature erythroid precursor (lower left). Although PAS-positive erythroblasts may be found in only small numbers in MDSs, progression to an erythroleukemia would be manifested by increased numbers of PAS-positive erythroid precursors. BM (×1,000).

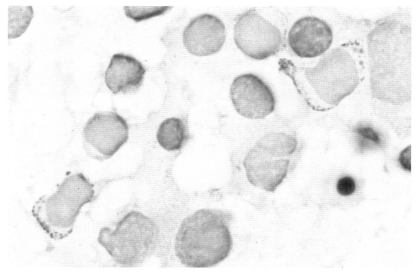

Figure 4.3b Bone marrow aspirate from a patient with large granular lymphocyte disease that may mimic an MDS. PAS reaction shows granules at the periphery of the lymphoid cells on a clear background (lower left and upper right) similar to the staining pattern in some acute lymphoblastic leukemias (×1,000).

marrow fibrosis seem to represent a distinct clinicopathological entity which has an unfavorable prognosis primarily attributable to complications deriving from pancytopenia and continuous transfusions; by contrast, leukemic transformation occurs rarely. These patients show cluster blastic infiltration and megakaryocytic hyperplasia, in contrast to those with large blastic infiltration, which is associated with a high percentage of leukemic transformation and a poor prognosis. By contrast, secondary MDS with extensive fibrosis represents a variety of preleukemic conditions in subjects treated for previous neoplasias. Unlike the primary forms, they do not form a clear-cut clinicopathological entity.

A bone marrow specimen of a patient with secondary MDS stained for reticulin appears in Fig. 3.5 in Chapter 3.

MASSON'S TRICHROME STAIN

Masson's trichrome stain, a histochemical reaction, is used in bone marrow biopsy sections to evaluate the presence of true collagen fibrosis. With this stain, nuclei are black and cytoplasm, keratin, muscle fibers, trabecular bone, and intracellular fibrils are stained red. Importantly, true collagen fibers are stained either blue or light green.

The probable mechanism of action is dependent upon the production of hematein lakes which result from an oxidation product of hematoxylin. The nuclear staining is ensured by the hematein lakes; consequently, intracellular structures become much clearer. The cytoplasm is stained with Biebrich scarlet. Then, treatment with phosphomolybdic acid uncoats the collagen fibers, which are stained with aniline blue.

Mild to moderate myelofibrosis has been reported in up to 50% of MDS patients. However, the occurrence of marked fibrosis (positive Masson trichrome stain) complicating the course of myelodysplasia is much lower (11–15%). Nevertheless, the incidence of myelofibrosis in t-MDS is consistently greater than that seen in primary MDS. Mild fibrosis occurs in up to 85% and marked fibrosis in up to 50% of t-MDS cases. Fibrosis has been evaluated on a 1 to 4+ scale, with 1 to 2+ being mild to moderate, 3+ moderately severe (negative collagen stain), and 4+ severe (positive collagen stain). The bone marrow specimens described in patients with MDS and fibrosis revealed that the majority were classified as either 3+ or 4+. A Masson trichrome stain is shown in Fig. 4.4.

MYELOPEROXIDASE (MPEX)

Originally, the MPEX stain employed benzidine dihydrochloride, which permitted transfer of hydrogen ions from the benzidine to hydrogen peroxide, leaving a black derivative of the dye. Since benzidine is well known for its carcinogenicity, alternative chromogens have been utilized. These include o-toluidine-3 amino-9-ethylcarbazole, Hanker-Yates reagent (p-phenylenediamine and pyrocatechol), and 4-chloro-1-naphthol. We use 4-chloro-1-naphthol as a chromogen and May-Grunwald-Giemsa as a counterstain. This is superior to the older technique that

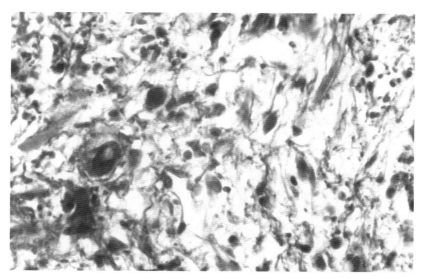

Figure 4.4   Bone marrow biopsy specimen stained with Masson trichrome stain in a patient with RAEB-IT. This represents true collagen and usually develops after precollagen, as demonstrated by reticulin stain. Note the trapped megakaryocytes ($\times 400$).

used methyl green counterstain. Myeloperoxidase activity is found in the primary granules of the granulocytic series and in the lysosomal granules of the monocytic series. Myeloblasts may or may not stain with MPEX at the light microscopic level, but may show staining of the perinuclear cisternae and endoplasmic reticulum prior to packaging into granules at the transmission electron microscopy level.

MPEX activity of neutrophilic granulocytes during the course of MDS has been reported to be significantly reduced. This reduction may be manifested by an increase in the percentage of MPEX-negative neutrophilic granulocytes or by an obvious decrease in the average content of MPEX in all granulocytes.

More than 4% MPEX-negative granulocytes have been observed in all subtypes of MDS. Apparently, a significant increase in the percentage of MPEX-negative granulocytes in the course of MDS is associated with a greater risk of disease progression and may be regarded as a potentially unfavorable prognostic factor. However, this event may not be an unavoidable step in such a progression.

MDS patients with a decrease in the average content of MPEX in all granulocytes do not show leukemic transformation, but they do have an increased incidence of infectious episodes. This may be related either to the reduced MPEX content in the granulocytes or to abnormal consumption of MPEX secondary to repeated infectious episodes caused by cytopenias.

Recently, Koni and Chiba (1992) evaluated 19 MDS patients, using the Technicon H-1 system, and observed that the mean peroxidase activity index was significantly low at the time of diagnosis and declined at the terminal stage in cases of death with bone marrow failure. A scattergram showing MPEX activity in MDS patient is depicted in Fig. 4.5.

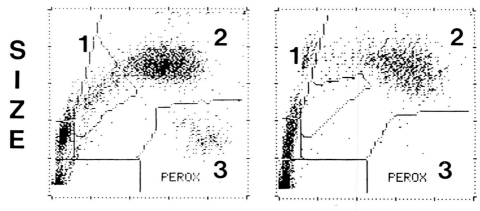

PEROXIDASE ACTIVITY

Figure 4.5 A myeloperoxidase histogram of a normal control (left) and a patient with RAEB (right) from a Technicon H-1 automated blood analyzer. Note that all of the neutrophils are positive for myeloperoxidase in area 2 of the normal control. By contrast, the RAEB patient shows a small population of myeloperoxidase-deficient cells in area 1. Note that many myeloperoxidase-positive cells remain in area 2. (Courtesy of Thomas Panke.)

NAPHTHOL AS-D CHLOROACETATE ESTERASE (CAE)

The CAE enzyme is specific for cells of the granulocytic series, with some exceptions. However, the stain is less sensitive than MPEX in demonstrating that leukemic blasts are of myeloid origin. This is most likely because CAE usually begins accumulating in the promyelocytic stage. The esterase reaction is initiated when blood and bone marrow films are incubated with naphthol AS-D chloroacetate in the presence of a stable diazonium salt. Enzymatic hydrolysis of ester linkage liberates free naphthol compounds. These couple with the diazonium salt to form highly colored deposits at the sites of enzyme activity.

Although CAE has been used in some studies of MDS patients, it seems to be of more value when employed in the combined esterase staining procedure. Results with CAE alone seems to parallel those obtained with the MPEX stain in MDS. A CAE stain of a bone marrow specimen from a patient with RAEB showing abnormal features is depicted in Fig. 4.6.

NONSPECIFIC ESTERASES (NSE)

NSE are enzymes that hydrolyze several synthetic substrates, showing strong positivity in monocytes and weaker or negative activity in other normal or pathological cells. The nonspecific substrates used are usually alpha naphthyl acetate and alpha naphthyl butyrate. The esterase activity may be detected in leukocytes when either of these substrates is used along with appropriate dye couplers. We use fast blue RR for A-EST detection, which produces a punctate black reaction

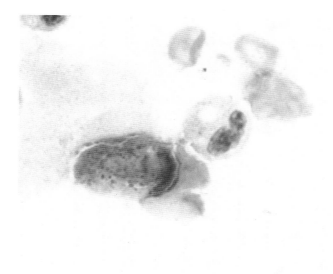

Figure 4.6 Bone marrow aspirate from a patient with RAEB stained with chloracetate esterase. Note the asynchrony in staining, i.e., the immature granulocytic element is strongly positive, and the band is negative for the staining product (×1,000).

product, and pararosaniline for B-EST, which yields a diffuse reddish-brown stain. A-EST appears to be more sensitive and less specific than B-EST. Sodium fluoride may be used to inhibit the A-EST reaction and make the procedure more specific for monocytic cells. Both A-EST and B-EST are invaluable in evaluating cells of the monocytic series. For this reason, they are of use in CMML and in those MDSs that are evolving toward an acute monomyelocytic or monocytic leukemia. They are best utilized in MDS when combined with CAE in the combined esterase stain (see below). Since A-EST is strongly positive in megakaryocytes and since B-EST is either negative or weakly positive, they can be considered presumptive evidence for megakaryocytic lineage.

COMBINED ESTERASE (C-EST)

A C-EST using both CAE and A-EST (or B-EST) has been employed in most laboratories to evaluate both the monocytic and granulocytic series on the same slide. Therefore, it is very helpful in diagnosing CMML. The presence of both CAE and the NSEs has been observed in myeloid precursor cells in acute leukemias and in primary and secondary MDS (hybrid cells). Seo et al. (1993) observed that of 70 of their 107 cases of primary and secondary MDS with ringed sideroblasts, 56 cases (80%) had dysplastic hybrid cells. These findings confirmed those of Scott et al. (1983), who noted that sideroblastosis is associated with a substantial increase in hybrid cells in cases of MDS. Apparently, MDS cases demonstrate more combined esterase-positive cells than do cases of non-MDS hematological disorders or nondiagnostic control marrows. Although overlap may exist, the cells of the

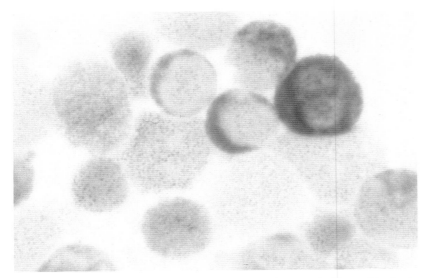

Figure 4.7 Bone marrow aspirate from a patient with RAEB-IT stained with combined esterase (C-EST). Note that the cells at the lower left stain with A-EST (small black dots), whereas those in the upper right stain red with CAE. Some CAE-positive cells also contain small black granules due to additional A-EST staining (hybrid cells) (×1,000).

non-MDS groups never exceed 10% combined esterase positivity. A C-EST stain on a MDS patient is shown in Fig. 4.7.

LEUKOCYTE ALKALINE PHOSPHATASE (LAP)

The precise function and subcellular localization of LAP in neutrophils remain unclear. LAP is a zinc-containing phosphomonoesterase with a pH optimum near 10 that catalyzes the hydrolysis of a wide variety of phosphoester substances. The activity of LAP, which is limited to the granulocytic series, first appears in myelocytes and rapidly increases with maturation of the cell to the neutrophil stage.

Most techniques for evaluation of LAP use an azo dye coupling procedure, employing a substituted naphthol compound as the substrate and fast violet B or fast blue RR salt as a coupler. Fresh peripheral blood and/or bone marrow may be stained, and a reaction product is observed within the neutrophils. The slides are counterstained with hematoxylin.

The majority of studies evaluating LAP activity in MDS have been devoted to the analysis of circulating neutrophils. The results reported have been quite erratic, since different cases may show increased, reduced, or normal enzyme content, with no precise correlation with different cytological variants of MDS. Nevertheless, some authors believe that a reduction in LAP activity does have some diagnostic value. Such low enzyme values can usually be distinguished from other diseases (i.e., CML, paroxysmal hemoglobinuria, some cases of AML, hypophosphatemia, and infectious mononucleosis).

Further information may be obtained by applying the LAP stain to bone marrow. Normally, the enzyme activity of bone marrow neutrophilic granulocytes is noticeably lower than that of circulating cells. However, rare cases of RA with normal LAP scores in the peripheral blood show a marked increase in the number of positive bone marrow cells. Contrariwise, all cases with low LAP scores in the peripheral blood reveal bone marrow granulocytes that are completely negative, suggesting the existence of an intrinsic metabolic defect.

In addition to LAP alteration in the granulocytic series, rare cases of pathological activity of alkaline phosphatase have been observed in proerythroblasts in a case of RA and in dysmorphic megakaryocytes in two cases of RA.

TERMINAL DEOXYNUCLEOTIDYL TRANSFERASE (Tdt)

Tdt is an unusual deoxynucleotide-polymerizing enzyme that catalyzes the addition of deoxynucleotide triphosphate to the 3'-hydroxyl ends of the oligo- and polydeoxynucleotides without template instruction. Its presence has been evaluated by indirect immunofluorescent and immunoperoxidase procedures. It has also been evaluated by flow cytometry. Although it has been an invaluable marker in the acute leukemias and in blast crisis of CML, Tdt is known to be positive in MDS cases with early B-lymphoid and mixed biphenotypic lineages. These findings support the concept that in a significant proportion of patients with MDS, the blast population corresponds to early precursors, showing immunophenotypical features characteristic of myeloid and lymphoid lineages. The prognostic implications of Tdt + MDS have not been explored.

IMMUNOCYTOHISTOCHEMISTRY

Background

Surface marker analysis of cell lineage in the diagnosis of the acute leukemias has been applied to the diagnosis and understanding of the MDSs. However, the immunophenotypic characteristics of blast cells in the MDSs have been poorly investigated due to the cell heterogeneity and low proportion of blasts usually present in blood and/or bone marrow. To overcome these difficulties, some investigators have employed immunoalkaline phosphatase techniques to perform immunocytochemistry, and others have used immunoperoxidase techniques to carry out immunohistochemistry.

Myeloid Phenotypes

The most common myeloid phenotypes are CD13+, CD14+, CD33+, and peroxidase +. San et al. (1991) evaluated acute leukemias following a previous primary MDS and found that although the granulocytic and/or monocytic lineages are most commonly involved, other cell components, including the megakaryocytic and lymphoid lineages, may also be present. Moreover, they observed that both morphological and phenotypic studies showed frequent coexistence of two or

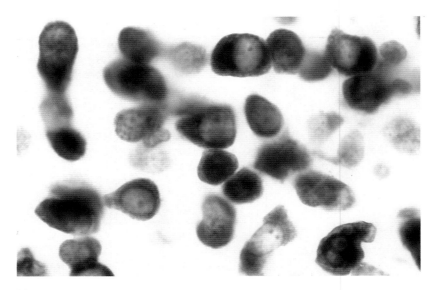

Figure 4.8 Bone marrow biopsy specimen from a patient with AML after bone marrow transplantation showing ALIP by antiperoxidase-immunoperoxidase technique. Cells are myeloblasts, which should not normally be observed in this location (×1,000).

three cell populations. They further noted that RAEB and RAEB-IT displayed a significantly higher incidence of myeloblastic transformation, whereas RA, RARS, and CMML demonstrated a granulomonocytic phenotype. Immunohistochemical studies have been performed on formalin-fixed, paraffin-embedded bone marrow biopsy specimens by Mangi and Mufti (1992) to discern the nature of ALIP. Three types of ALIP were identified: erythroid, megakaryocytic, and granulocytic-monocytic aggregates. The authors conclude that the term *abnormal localization of immature precursors* should be applied only to those cases in which the clusters in the intertrabecular region are of granulocytic-monocytic lineage on immunohistochemistry. The term *pseudo–abnormal localization of immature precursors* has been applied to megakaryocytic and erythroid aggregates by some authors. ALIP are depicted in Fig. 4.8.

Lymphoid Phenotype

Early B-lymphoid phenotypes (CD19+, CD10−, Tdt+) and more differentiated forms (CD19+, CD10+, Tdt+) have been reported. Apparently, those primary MDSs that develop into acute leukemia have a pluripotent stem cell with a preferential myeloid commitment as the target cell. This finding has been supported by Guyotat et al. (1990), who observed that CD34 (stem cell/myeloid differentiation) was expressed in those RAEB and RAEB-IT patients who showed early progression to leukemia and shorter survival. The presence of CD34 has also been associated with poor survival in AML.

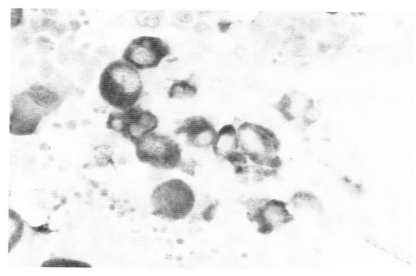

Figure 4.9 Bone marrow biopsy specimen from a patient after bone marrow transplantation for CML in blastic crisis. The anti-factor VIII-immunoperoxidase technique was utilized. Note the large numbers of clustered immature megakaryocytes (pseudo ALIP) (×400).

Mixed-Biphenotypic Phenotypes

Besides myeloid, lymphoid, and stem cell/myeloid phenotypic expression in MDS, mixed phenotypes have been reported. Some have been B-lymphoid and myeloid (CD19+, CD13+, CD14+, Tdt+, α-peroxidase+); others T-lymphoid and myeloid (CD3+, CD2+, Tdt+, α-peroxidase+); and still others have shown B- and T-lymphoid, as well as myeloid markers (CD19+, CD10+, CD3+, CD2+, CD13+, Tdt+).

Megakaryocytic Phenotype

Immunological techniques have been applied to the characterization of dysmega-karyopoiesis in the bone marrow of MDS patients by the alkaline phosphatase anti-alkaline phosphatase (APAAP) technique. In dysmegakaryopoiesis, abnormally small megakaryoblasts may resemble lymphoid precursors similar to FAB L-2 lymphoblasts. Monoclonal antibodies to gp IIb/IIIa (CD41), gp Ib (CD42b), or gp IIIa(CD61) have been used to identify these abnormal megakaryocytic precursors. In addition, antibodies to platelet gp IIb, factor VIII–related antigen, and fibronec-tin have been used to document megakaryocytic lineage in otherwise ambiguous cells. The APAAP not only markedly increased the ability to classify correctly abnormal megakaryocytes in the marrow, but also made it possible to identify megakaryoblasts. Besides the APAAP technique for identification of megakaryo-cytic series on air-dried slides, immunoperoxidase techniques employing an anti-body against factor VIII may be utilized (Fig. 4.9).

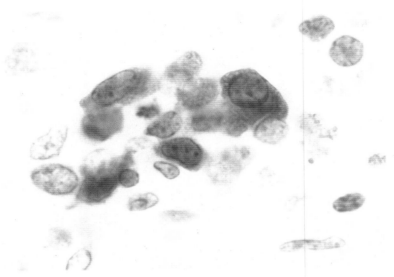

Figure 4.10 Bone marrow biopsy specimen from a patient with AML after bone marrow transplantation demonstrating pseudo-ALIP. The anti-hemoglobin immunoperoxidase method was used. Note the immature clusters of erythroid elements (×400).

Erythroid Phenotype

Erythroid progenitors may be identified by antibodies to glycophorin A, transferrin receptor (CD71), and HLe-1 (CD45). Immunophenotyping is especially helpful in those cases in which ringed sideroblasts are absent and PAS staining is equivocal or negative. HLe-1 (CD45) is expressed on the earliest identifiable erythroid cells and is progressively lost as cells undergo maturation. The transferrin receptor (CD71) is expressed during the erythroid burst-forming unit (BFU-E) stage and disappears in the late reticulocyte stage. Both HLe-1 (CD45) and the transferrin receptor (CD71) markers precede that of glycophorin. Glycophorin appears on morphologically recognizable erythroblasts just beyond the erythroid colony-forming unit (CFU-E) stage. Both HLe-1 (CD45) and transferrin receptor (CD71) are progressively lost during maturational development. In contrast, once glycophorin is maximally expressed on the cell surface, it remains fixed in quantity throughout the mature erythroid stage.

Antibodies to glycophorin A have been used to diagnose myelodysplastic cases that progressed to erythroleukemia. Of 20 cases of erythroleukemia described by Cuneo et al. (1990), 8 evolved from an initial MDS involving multiple hematopoietic lineages. Those patients with major karyotypic aberrations (MAKA) (three or more aberrant events in the same clone) were observed in 14 cases. Surprisingly, all patients with MAKA had a leftward shift in erythropoiesis, with proerythroblasts and basophilic erythroblasts usually representing more than 50% of all erythroid cells. By current FAB criteria, such cases are often diagnosed as MDS due to lack of sufficient numbers of myeloblasts. In fact, these cases represent pure erythroleukemia (Di Guglielmo's disease) and should so be diagnosed.

In our laboratory, we have had more success using an antibody to hemoglobin than glycophorin A with the immunoperoxidase technique. Interestingly, immature erythroid precursors containing hemoglobin can be demonstrated. A pseudo-ALIP is shown in Fig. 4.10.

BIBLIOGRAPHY

Articles

Bendix-Hansen K, Kerndrup G: Myeloperoxidase-deficient polymorphonuclear leukocytes V: Relation to FAB classification and neutrophil alkaline phosphatase activity in primary myelodysplastic syndromes. *Scand J Haematol* 35:197–200, 1985.

Choate JJ, Domenico DR, McGraw TP, et al: Diagnosis of acute megakaryoblastic leukemia by flow cytometry and immunoalkaline phosphatase techniques: Utilization of new monoclonal antibodies. *Am J Clin Pathol* 89:247–253, 1987.

Cuneo A, Van-Orshoven A, Michaux JL, et al: Morphologic, immunologic, and cytogenetic studies in erythroleukaemia: Evidence for multilineage involvement and identification of two distinct cytogenetic-clinicopathological types. *Br J Haematol* 75:346–354, 1990.

Doe KA, Gryzbac M, Schumacher HR: A new modified rapid noncarcinogenic myeloperoxidase staining technique using 4-chloro-1-naphthol. *Lab Med* 19:374–375, 1988.

Geller RB, Zahurak M, Hurwitz CA, et al: Prognostic importance of immunophenotyping in adults with acute myelocytic leukaemia: The significance of the stem-cell glycoprotein CD34 (My 10). *Br J Haematol* 76:340–347, 1990.

Grasso JA, Myers TJ, Hines JD, et al: Energy-dispersive X-ray analysis of the mitochondria of sideroblastic anaemia. *Br J Haematol* 46:57–72, 1980.

Guyotat D, Campos L, Thomas X, et al: Myelodysplastic syndromes: A study of surface markers and in vitro growth patterns. *Am J Hematol* 34:26–31, 1990.

Kawaguchi M, Nehashi Y, Aizawa S, et al: Comparative study of immunocytochemical staining versus Giemsa stain for detecting dysmegakaryocytopoiesis in myelodysplastic syndromes (MDS). *Eur J Haematol* 44:89–94, 1990.

Koni F, Chiba T: The clinicopathological evaluation of automated cytochemical hematology system (Technicon H-I) in patients with leukemia and myelodysplastic syndrome. *Rhinsko Byori* 40:586–594, 1992.

Kowal-Vern A, Cotelingam J, Schumacher HR: The prognostic significance of proerythroblasts in acute erythroleukemia. *Am J Clin Pathol* 98:34–40, 1992.

Loken MR, Shah VO, Dattilio KL, et al: Flow cytometric analysis of human bone marrow: I. Normal erythroid development. *Blood* 69:255–263, 1987.

Mangi MH, Mufti GJ: Primary myelodysplastic syndromes: Diagnostic and prognostic significance of immunohistochemical assessment of bone marrow biopsies. *Blood* 79:198–205, 1992.

Matutes E, Urbano-Ispizua A, Feliu E, et al: Immunophenotypical features of blast cells in myelodysplastic syndromes. *Blood* 72:215a, 1988.

Tham KT, Cousar JB, Macon WR: Silver stain for ringed sideroblasts: A sensitive method that differs from Perls' reaction in mechanism and clinical application. *Am J Clin Pathol* 94:73–76, 1990.

Thiele J, Quitman H, Wagner S, et al: Dysmegakaryopoiesis in myelodysplastic syndromes (MDS): An immunomorphometric study of bone marrow trephine biopsy specimens. *J Clin Pathol* 44:300–305, 1991.

Thiele J, Titius BR, Kopsidis C, et al: Atypical micromegakaryocytes, promegakary-oblasts, and megakaryoblasts: A critical evaluation by immunohistochemistry, cytochemistry and morphometry of bone marrow trephines in chronic myeloid leukemia and myelodysplastic syndromes. *Virchows Arch B Cell Pathol* 62:275–282, 1992.

Review Articles

De Pasquale A, Quaglino D: Enzyme cytochemical studies in myelodysplastic syndromes. In Schmalzl F, Mufti GJ (eds): *Myelodysplastic Syndromes.* Berlin, Springer-Verlag, 1992, pp 51–59.

Hayhoe FG, Quaglimo D: *Haematological Cytochemistry,* ed 2. Edinburgh, Churchill Livingstone, 1988.

Kass L: *Leukemia: Cytology and Cytochemistry.* Philadelphia, JB Lippincott, 1982.

San Miguel JF, Hernandez JM, Gonzalez-Sarmiento R, et al: Acute leukemia after a primary myelodysplastic syndrome: Immunophenotypic, genotypic, and clinical characteristics. *Blood* 78:768–774, 1991.

Schmalzl F: The value of cytochemical investigations in the diagnosis of the myelodysplastic syndromes. In Schmalzl F, Mufti GJ (eds): *Myelodysplastic Syndromes.* Berlin, Springer-Verlag, 1992, pp 44–50.

Schumacher HR: *Acute Leukemia: Approach to Diagnosis.* New York, Igaku-Shoin, 1990, pp 33–50.

Schumacher HR, Cotelingam JD: *Chronic Leukemia: Approach to Diagnosis.* New York, Igaku-Shoin, 1993, pp 63–81.

Scott CS, Cahill A, Bynoe AG, et al: Esterase cytochemistry in primary myelodys-plastic syndromes and megaloblastic anaemias: Demonstration of abnormal staining patterns associated with dysmyelopoiesis. *Br J Haematol* 55:411–418, 1983.

Seo S, Li C-Y, Yam LT: Myelodysplastic syndrome: Diagnostic implications of cytochemical and immunocytochemical studies. *Mayo Clin Proc* 68:47–53, 1993.

Sun T, Li C-Y, Yam LT: *Atlas of Cytochemistry and Immunohistochemistry of Hemato-logic Neoplasms.* Chicago: American Society of Clinical Pathologists Press, 1985.

Third MIC Cooperative Study Group: Recommendations for a morphologic, im-munologic and cytogenetic (MIC) working classification of the primary and therapy-related myelodysplastic disorders: Report of the workshop held in Scottsdale, Arizona, USA, on February 23–25, 1987. *Cancer Genet Cytogenet* 32:1–10, 1988.

Woessner S, Lafuente R, Florensa L, et al: Cytochemical detection of erythroblastic enzymes in acquired dyserythropoiesis. *Acta Haematol* 72:303–308, 1984.

CHAPTER **5**

Transmission Electron Microscopy

INTRODUCTION

Although transmission electron microscopy (TEM) has not been necessary in the diagnosis of most cases of acute and chronic leukemias or in the myelodysplastic syndromes, it has been of great value in the difficult cases in which light microscopy, cytochemistry, immunohistochemistry, flow cytometry, cytogenetic analysis, and gene rearrangement analysis do not provide essential information for diagnosis. Recently, TEM has played an even more important role in such cases because of technological advances in specimen preparation. What formerly required several days now takes only a few hours. Since it is imperative for the clinician to obtain the correct diagnosis as quickly as possible to institute appropriate therapy, TEM has become an integral part of the diagnosis in some cases.

TEM has been of greatest value in those most difficult cases in which the diagnosis cannot be established with certainty. Some findings, such as Auer rods, bull's eyes, and basophilic and eosinophilic granules, clearly define the myeloid nature of the evolving leukemic process. Bull's-eye granules are associated with the monocytic and megakaryocytic leukemias and demonstrate a lucid area around the central granule. Ultrastructural MPEX staining is of great value in defining MDS with undifferentiated myeloid blasts. Ultrastructural platelet peroxidase can also be of value in clearly defining an immature megakaryocytic element in a MDS. Further, rhopheocytosis, an engulfment of ferritin by erythroblasts, may be used to identify immature erythroid precursors.

It is well known that clustering of blasts in the intertrabecular region in the

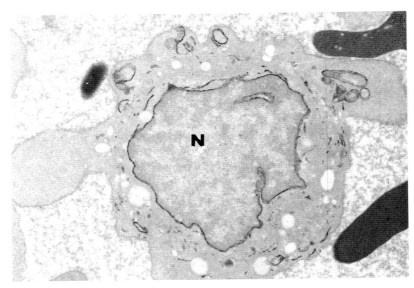

Figure 5.2   TEM of a megakaryoblast from a case of megakaryocytic leukemia specially fixed and stained for platelet peroxidase activity. The nucleus is somewhat irregular, with finely dispersed chromatin. Electron-dense deposits, indicating peroxidase activity, are seen in the perinuclear cistern and in short segments of endoplasmic reticulum. No granules are present. Two peripheral blebs are seen on either side. Adjacent red blood cells also show dark reaction products because of the peroxidase activity of hemoglobin (×16,000). (Courtesy of Raoul Fresco.)

and the Anderson technique (tannic acid/paraformaldehyde/glutaraldehyde) use diaminobenzidine as the electron-dense peroxidase stain. This stain is localized in the endoplasmic reticulum and the perinuclear space of early megakaryoblasts. It is distinct from granulocyte peroxidase because it is absent in the Golgi apparatus and granules. Both immunofluorescent and immunoalkaline phosphatase techniques, using monoclonal antibodies to platelet gp Ib (CD42b), IIb/IIIa (CD41), and IIIa (CD61), have been used to identify megakaryocytic precursors. Furthermore, histological bone marrow reaction with an antibody against factor VIII may be utilized. These techniques have an advantage over TEM-PPO detection for routine diagnosis of acute megakaryocytic leukemia or pseudomegakaryocytic ALIP in a MDS because of their simplicity compared to TEM-PPO. However, some combined studies employing both TEM-PPO and immunological staining for megakaryoblast surface gp have revealed that TEM-PPO positivity can be detected earlier than the IIb/IIIa complex by immunoalkaline phosphatase. The TEM-PPO staining reaction is demonstrated in Fig. 5.2.

Although proerythroblasts can usually be identified by Romanowsky stains and monoclonal antibodies, sometimes classification can be extremely difficult. Iida et al. (1991) have described a case with blast cells that were negative for lymphocytic, myelocytic, megakaryocytic, and erythrocytic markers but that had characteristic features of immature erythroblasts by electron microscopy. The patient responded poorly to low dose Ara-C therapy and expired from gastrointestinal hemorrhage. As can be concluded from the authors' description, this patient had pure erythroleukemia (Di Guglielmo's disease), in contrast to FAB M6, which

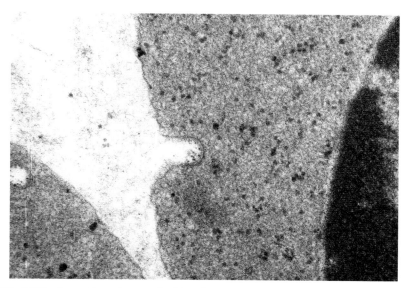

Figure 5.3 TEM of a portion of an erythroblast from a patient with erythroleukemia. The nucleus is to the right. A pinocytotic invagination of the cell membrane shows numerous small, dense ferritin particles (rhopheocytosis) (×125,000). (Courtesy of Raoul Fresco.)

represents Di Guglielmo's syndrome. We propose the latter be designated FAB M6A and the former M6B.

Erythroid precursors in MDS and erythroleukemia can be characterized at the ultrastructural level by examining unstained sections. Erythroid elements demonstrate rhopheocytosis, a phenomenon characterized by electron microscopic thickening and invagination of the cell membrane associated with electron-dense ferritin particles. The ferritin particles attach themselves to the membrane, and the invagination continues until a vacuole containing ferritin is pinched off. Next, the vacuole migrates into the cytoplasm and the ferritin is released. By electron microscopy, increased ferruginous micelles are deposited within the mitochondria encircling the nucleus and thus forming the pathological ringed sideroblast. Ringed sideroblasts may be found in any of the MDSs, but are increased to 15% or more of the erythroid population in patients with RARS and are frequently found in large numbers in patients with erythroleukemia. Rhopheocytosis, the ultrastructural finding identifying the erythroid series, is depicted in Fig. 5.3.

Besides assisting in identifying various cell types, as exemplified above, TEM may aid in characterizing cells in unusual cases of MDS, in describing unique morphological findings, or in detecting viruses in peculiar lesions.

Caldwell et al. (1990) used TEM to delineate more clearly a plasmacytoid T-cell leukemia/lymphoma occurring in a patient with long-standing MDS. The tumor demonstrated ultrastructural features consistent with a spectrum of plasmacytoid differentiation. Rare primitive-appearing cells showed dispersed central nucleoli, euchromatic nuclei, and cytoplasm containing free ribosomes, infrequent mitochondria, and rare lysosomes. Approximately 10% of the tumor cells displayed well-developed plasma cell features with peripheral condensations of chromatin, prominent cytoplasmic arrays of focally dilated rough endoplasmic

marrow specimens with the findings of MDS revealed frequent large tubuloreticular structures in lymphocytes, plasma cells, macrophages, and endothelial cells.

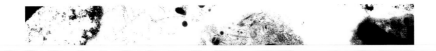

progression to leukemia and shorter survival. Furthermore, they suggested that surface marker analysis at the time of diagnosis and after liquid culture may be useful for the initial evaluation of MDS.

Besides the use of lymphoid and myeloid monoclonal antibodies, immunological techniques have been applied to the characterization of megakaryocytes in MDSs. In dysmegakaryocytopoiesis, the abnormally small megakaryoblasts (dwarf cells) may resemble lymphoid precursors similar to FAB L2 lymphoblasts. These cells can be easily identified on air-dried smears with an antibody prepared against platelet-specific gp IIb/IIIa (CD41), gp Ib (CD42b), or gp IIIa (CD61) by alkaline phosphatase anti-alkaline phosphatase technique or by immunohistochemical bone marrow reaction with an antibody against factor VIII. Monoclonal antibodies to glycophorin A, the transferrin receptor (CD71), and leukocyte common antigen (LCA; CD45) can be useful in identifying erythroid progenitors. The latter reactions have permitted analysis of erythroid maturation from colony-forming cells to the mature erythrocyte.

As mentioned above, due to the paucity of cells, surface marker analysis in the MDSs has not been easily accomplished by flow cytometric analysis unless evolution to acute leukemia has occurred. However, immunocytochemistry and immunofluorescent techniques have been successfully employed to determine cell lineage in the MDSs. Immunocytochemical staining methods may be applied to sections of fresh frozen tissue, touch preparations, aspirates, and paraffin-embedded tissues. Immunofluorescence can also be utilized on all these preparations, with the exception of paraffin-embedded material. Both immunocytochemical and immunofluorescent techniques have the advantage of direct cell and/or tissue analysis and relatively low-budget operation. Furthermore, they allow the hematopathologist to examine the cells in relation to total tissue architecture. Therefore, these techniques are ideally suited for small biopsy specimens and for specimens that are only focally involved with disease, as seen in the MDSs. The disadvantages of these techniques include slow, tedious analysis and some lack of objectivity and reproducibility. Careful analysis of specimens for staining artifacts and controls are imperative. Flow cytometric analysis on those cases of MDSs that have enough cells for evaluation or that have evolved to acute leukemia has the following advantages: fast analysis, objectivity, reproducibility, estimation of cell size and granularity, simultaneous measurement of different markers by multicolored analysis fluorescence, sensitivity of small subpopulation detection, accurate quantitation of fluorescence intensity, and good documentation of data. It suffers, however, from the following disadvantages: high cost of instrumentation and the training of operators, loss of tissue and architecture orientation, and occasional difficulty in sorting and obtaining single-cell suspensions. Also, cytospins need to be examined to determine the morphology of the populations analyzed. The parameters of positivity in flow cytometry vary from laboratory to laboratory, but depend on the intensity of fluorescence and the number of positive cells seen with a particular monoclonal antibody. Additionally, a caveat associated with any test is that the specimens evaluated must obviously contain the appropriate material for analysis. In general, values less than 30% positivity for single-color analyses within a given cell population (gate) are not considered significant. However, with two- and three-color analysis, this percentage can be lowered to 5–10%.

In addition to immunophenotypic cellular variation in MDSs, patients with

MDSs clearly have disordered immune systems. Mufti et al. (1986) observed that infections accounted for at least one-fifth of all deaths. Since most patients have neutropenia and/or granulocytic dysfunction, it would be easy to presume that the infections result from a disordered effector function and that the central immune system is intact. However, further investigation has demonstrated a wide range of immunological abnormalities in patients with MDSs. Currently, whether these abnormalities are primary, incriminating the lymphoid system within the dysplastic clone, and/or secondary to an abnormality of granulocyte/macrophage function requires additional exploration.

IMMUNOPHENOTYPE

Although the analysis of cell surface antigens is widely used in the diagnosis of acute leukemias, limitations exist in the MDSs due to lack of cells for analysis and cell heterogeneity. Nevertheless, Matutes et al. (1988) have applied an immunoalkaline phosphatase technique to study blast cells from 20 MDS cases (6-RAEB, 9-RAEB-IT, and 5-CMML). The myeloid immunophenotype of these cases was CD13+, CD68+, CD14+/−, and α-peroxidase positive in 15 cases; in 1 of them, the blasts showed basophilic differentiation by ultrastructural analysis. Other studies on bone marrow samples from patients with RAEB and RAEB-IT showed less mature myeloid phenotypes (low percentages of CD24-positive cells). These blasts expressed HLA-DR, CDw65, CD13, and CD33 antigens, whereas some of the blast cells in RAEB-IT patients reacted with an anti-H antibody (of the O_h blood group). The number of H substance (or antigen)-positive blasts was much lower in RAEB, representing particularly erythroid precursors. Anti-H antibody is specific for involvement of the erythroid/megakaryocytic lineage and thus indicates a mixed lineage phenotype. The presence of blast cells in AML expressing H antigen indicates a poor prognosis; therefore, MDS patients expressing this antigen may also fare poorly.

Investigation of patients with AML following primary MDS with abnormalities of chromosome 5q revealed an immature myeloid phenotype (CDw65, CD13+, CD33+) and reactivity with the anti-H antibody suggesting a mixed myeloid/erythroid lineage phenotype. Mixed biphenotypic (myeloid and lymphoid) lineages were observed in four cases. Two were B-lymphoid and myeloid, demonstrating Tdt+, CD19+, CD13+, CD14+, and α-peroxidase positivity. The other two cases were myeloid and T-lymphoid, expressing Tdt+, CD2+, CD3+, CD13+, and α-peroxidase + immunophenotypic features. Recently, a study by Reading et al. (1993) evaluating by two-color immunofluorescence flow cytometric analysis the immunophenotypes of 272 patients with AML, revealed unusual coexpression of T-lymphoid, B-lymphoid, or NK cell markers with myeloid markers in 38%, 13%, and 21% of cases, respectively. Therefore, mixed immunophenotypes occur in both MDSs and the AMLs with some frequency. However, Matutes et al. (1988) were not able to detect the presence of megakaryoblastic (CD41) and/or erythroid (α-glycophorin A) positivity in any of their MDS cases evaluated by the immunoalkaline phosphatase technique. Koeller et al. (1992), in evaluating small numbers of RA and RARS patients by indirect immunofluorescence staining using a large

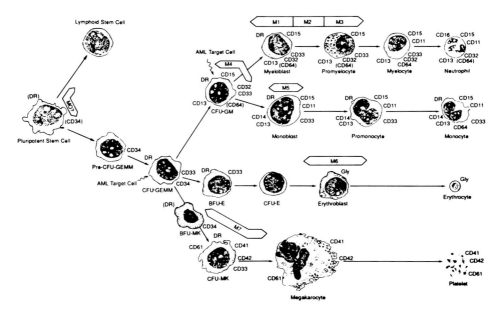

Figure 6.1 Hypothetical myeloid differentiation scheme indicating the cell surface markers—as defined by selected, well-characterized cluster designations (CDs)—that have been detected on cells at the various maturational stages, either by immunofluorescence, positive selection (sorting followed by colony forming unit [CFU] assay), or negative selection (complement-mediated lysis). Hypothetical target cells in AML are indicated by small, wavy arrows. Major phenotypic manifestations of the FAB subtypes (M0–M7) are in boxes. Parentheses around a CD marker indicate speculative placement (CD34, DR on a pluripotent stem cell), weak expression (CD64 on myeloid precursors), or inducibility (CD64 on a mature neutrophil). (From Vaickus L, Immune markers in hematologic malignancies. *CRC Crit Rev Oncol Hematol* 11:267–297, 1991.)

panel of myeloid monoclonal antibodies, were unable to demonstrate remarkable differences between the patient group and healthy controls. Nevertheless, one RA and one RARS patient showed slightly elevated numbers of CD13+ and CD33+ cells, which in one patient corresponded to elevated numbers of CD14+ monocytes. A schematic representation of human myeloid differentiation indicating the cell surface marker phenotype (as defined by well-characterized, selected monoclonal reagents) of identifiable maturational steps is depicted in Fig. 6.1. Table 6.1 shows the clinically used monoclonal antibodies for myeloid disorders. Although immunophenotyping currently is not of great importance in MDSs, it may become more significant as various treatment modalities evolve. A complete updated list of the cluster designation antigens is shown in Table 6.2. Note that this information is available in detail on computer disc from the National Institutes of Health.

Immunological techniques have also been applied to the characterization of megakaryocytes in MDS. Dysmegakaryocytopoiesis with abnormally small megakaryoblasts may resemble lymphoid precursors similar to FAB L2 lymphoblasts. These small blast cells have been identified on air-dried smears with an antibody prepared against platelet-specific gp IIb/IIIa (CD41a) by alkaline phosphatase anti-alkaline phosphatase technique. Using this technique (CD41a), Kawaguchi

Table 6.1 Clinically Used Myeloid Antibodies

Antibody	Specificity	Cluster Designation
MHM24; 2F12; CRIS-3; IDT16	Leukocytes	CD11a
M01; OKM1; I0M1	N, G, Nk	CD11b
B-LY6; L29; BL-4H4; I0M11c	M, G, Nk, B Sub	CD11c
M67; 20.2	G, M, Plt	CDw12
My7, MCS-2, 44H, I0M13	M, G	CD13
M02; My4; M3; FMC17; FMC 33; I0M2; UChM1; VIM13; M0p15	M, (G), LHC	CD14
My1; MCS1; Leu M1; VImD5; FMC10; OKM15; I0N1	G, (M)	CD15
GO35; Huly-m13	G, M, Plt	CDw17
MHM23; M232; 11H6; GLB54; I0T18; LFA1B	Leukocytes	CD18
CIKM5; 41H16; IV.3; 2E1, K361	M, G, B, Plt	CDw32
My9, H153; L4F3	M, G, Prog., AML	CD33
My10; HPCA 1; HPCA 2; 12.8; B1-3C; ICH 3 Q BEND-10	Prog.	CD34
My8	G, M	NA
Ep-1	E, BFU-E, CFU-E	NA
LICR, LON, R10	E, glycophorin A	NA
J15; 10E5; PBM 6.4; Plt 1; Pl 273; I0P41a	Plt GP IIb/IIIa	CD41a
I0P41b	Plt GP II b	CD41b
FMC25; BL-H6; GR-P; I042a	Plt GPIX, gp 23	CD42a
PHN89; 6D1, AN51; GN27; I0P42b	Plt GP Ib, gp 135/25	CD42b
Hle-1; T29/33; T-200; BMAC 1; AB187, I0L1a,b,c	Leucocytes	CD45
G1-15; F8-11-13; 73.5; I0L2; Leu 18; 2H4; CD45R	T subset, B, G, M	CD45A
PTD/26/16; CD45RB	T subset, B, G, M	CD45B
UCH1 1; IO13; Leu 45RO; CD45 RO	T subset, B, G, M	CD45RO

Abbreviations: M = monocytes; G = granulocytes; Nk = natural killer; ( ) = some; E = erythrocytes; N = neutrophils; Plt = platelets; NA = not applicable, no CD assigned, B sub = B subtype, LCH = epidermal Langerhans cell, Prog = progenitor cells.

et al. (1990) were able to detect dysmegakaryopoiesis in 91% (21/23) of MDS cases, whereas only 52% (12/123) were detectable by Giemsa staining. Also, Thiele et al. (1991), using a formalin-resistant monoclonal antibody against gp IIIa (CD61) on trephine biopsy specimens, were able to demonstrate dysmegakaryopoiesis and increased numbers of micromegakaryocytes in 31 of 40 patients studied.

Furthermore, immunohistochemical staining using factor VIII, VEA-1, gp IIa (CD31), and CD34 has been employed by Calapso et al. (1992) to identify atypical megakaryocytes and micromegakaryocytes in both MDSs and the myeloproliferative disorders.

Erythroid progenitors can be identified by an antibody to glycophorin A which may enhance understanding of the MDSs. Orazi et al. (1993) employed anti-glycophorin, CD34, anti-HLA-DR, CD68, CD61, and anti-elastase monoclonal anti-

Table 6.2b CD Antigens

CD Designation	Common Name	Workshop Section	MW Reduced	CD Designation	Common Name	Workshop Section	MW Reduced
CD15s	sLeˣ, Sialyl Lewisˣ	Adhesion		CD85	VMP-55, GH1/75	B cell	120, 83
CD16	FcR IIIA/FcR IIIB	Myeloid	50-65	CD86	FUN-1, BU63	B cell	80
CD16b	FcR IIIB	Myeloid	48	CD87	UPA-R	Myeloid	50-65
CD32	Previously CDw32, FcRII	Myeloid	40	CD88	C5aR	Myeloid	42
CD42a	GPIX	Platelets	23	CD89	FcαR	Myeloid	55-75
CD42b	GPIB, α	Platelets	135, 23	CDw90	Thy-1	Myeloid	25-35
CD42c	GP1B-β	Platelets	22	CD91	α$_2$M-R	Myeloid	600
CD42d	GPV	Platelets	85	CDw92		Myeloid	70
CD44	Pgp-1	Adhesion	80-90	CD93		Myeloid	120
CD44R	Restricted epitope on CD44	Adhesion		CD94	KP43	NK cell	43
CD49a	VLA-1, α1 integrin chain	Adhesion	210	CD95	APO-1, FAS	Activation	42
CD49b	VLA-2, α2 integrin chain	Adhesion	160	CD96	TACTILE	Activation	160
CD49c	VLA-3, α3 integrin chain	Adhesion	125	CD97		Activation	74, 80, 89
CD49d	VLA-4, α4 integrin chain	Adhesion	150, 80, 70	CD98	4F2, 2F3	T cell	80, 40
CD49e	VLA-5, α5 integrin chain	Adhesion	135, 25	CD99	E2, MIC2	T cell	32
CD49f	VLA-6, α6 integrin chain	Adhesion	120, 25	CD99R	CD99 mAb restricted	T cell	32
CD50	ICAM-3	Adhesion	124	CD100	BB18, A8	T cell	150
CD51/ CD61	Complex dependent epitope	Adhesion		CDw101	BB27, BA27	T cell	140
				CD102	ICAM-2	Adhesion	60

CD	Also known as	Category	MW (kD)
CD52	Campath-1	Blind	21–28
CD62E	E-selectin, ELAM-1	Adhesion	115
CD62L	L-selectin, LAM-1, TQ-1	Adhesion	75–80
CD62P	P-selectin, GMP-140, PADGEM	Adhesion	150
CD66a	BGP	Myeloid	180–200
CD66b	CD67, p100, CGM6	Myeloid	95–100
CD66c	NCA	Myeloid	90–95
CD66d	CGM1	Myeloid	30
CD66e	CEA, carcinoembryonic antigen	Myeloid	180–200
CD67	Now CD66b		
CD70	CD27-ligand	Activation	55, 75, 95, 110, 170
CDw76	Previously CD76	B cell	NA
CD79a	mb-1, Igα	B cell	33, 40
CD79b	B29, Igβ	B cell	33, 40
CD80	B7, BB1	B cell	60
CD81	TAPA-1	B cell	22
CD82	R2, IA4, 4F9	B cell	50–53
CD83		B cell	43
CDw84		B cell	73
CD103	HML-1	Adhesion	150, 25
CD104	β4 integrin chain	Adhesion	220
CD105	Endoglin	Endothelial	95
CD106	VCAM-1, INCAM-110	Endothelial	100, 110
CD107a	LAMP-1	Platelet	110
CD107b	LAMP-2	Platelet	120
CDw108		Adhesion	80
CDw109	8A3, 7D1	Endothelial	170/150
CD115	CSF-1R, M-CSFR	Myeloid	150
CDw116	HGM-CSFR, GM-CSFR	Cytokine	75–85
CD117	SCFR, cKIT	Cytokine	145
CDw119	IFNγR	Cytokine	90
CD120a	TNFR; 55kD	Cytokine	55
CD120b	TNFR; 75KD	Cytokine	75
CDw121a	IL-1R; Type 1	Cytokine	80
CDw121b	IL-1R; Type 2	Cytokine	68
CD122	IL-2R; 75KD, IL-2Rβ	Cytokine	75
CD124	IL-4R	Cytokine	140
CD126	IL-6R	Cytokine	80
CDw127	IL-7R	Cytokine	75
IL-8R	CDw128	Cytokine	58–67
CDw130	IL-GR-gp130SIG	Cytokine	130

Source: Schlossman SF, Boumsell L, Gilks W, et al: CD antigens 1993 (commentary). *Blood* 83:879–880. 1994. Reprinted with permission.
**Fifth International Workshop on Human Leukocyte Differentiation Antigens, Boston MA, November 3–7, 1993.
Leukocyte Differentiation Antigen Database Version 1.10, July 1994 available on computer disc. Stephen Shaw, National Institutes of Health.

Table 6.3 Key Immunological Abnormalities in the MDSs

Immunoglobulins
    Polyclonal hypergammaglobulinemia
    Hypogammaglobulinemia
    Monoclonal gammopathy
    Anti-red cell antibodies
B cells
    Normal in number
    Functionally immature
T cells
    T-cell lymphopenia
    Reduced CD4-positive cells
    Impaired T-cell function
NK cells
    Reduced in number
    Functionally immature
Monocytes
    Normal, reduced or increased numbers
    Impaired monocyte function

Source: Hamblin T: Immunologic abnormalities in myelodysplastic syndrome. *Hematol Oncol Clin North Am* 6:573, 1992.

using a panel of monoclonal antibodies to p-170 (C219, JSB1, C494, MRK16) and quantitative analysis of MDR-1 mRNA. Expression of p-170 was associated with the presence of blast cells characterized by an immature or early myeloid phenotype, as defined by CD34 co-expression with CD13 or CD33, or CD13/33 plus Tdt double expression. Expression of p-170 was present in 13/15 (86%) patient samples with an abnormal karyotype as compared with 3/10 (30%) samples with a normal karyotype. Therefore, the presence of CD34 positivity in MDSs is associated with shorter survival and progression to leukemia. Similarly shortened survival has been observed in those AMLs expressing CD34.

IMMUNOLOGICAL ABNORMALITIES (Table 6.3)

Infections

Infections are common in patients with MDS. Approximately 10% of all patients present with evidence of infection, and about 65% of all patient deaths are due to infection and/or hemorrhage. Infections most commonly occur in the lower respiratory tract, with rectal or perineal infections and bacterial sepsis accounting for most of the remainder. Although gram-negative septicemias and bacterial bronchopneumonias predominate, fungal and mycobacterial infections may occur. Even though infections with organisms characteristically observed in T-cell deficiencies such as *Pneumocystis carinii*, cytomegalovirus, *Cryptococcus neoformans*, or cryptosporidium are unusual, *Candida albicans* infections are common in MDS, especially in patients on antibiotic therapy. Recently, Shitara et al. (1993) have reported two cases of invasive aspergillosis in patients with leukemic transformation of a myelodysplastic syndrome.

Fungal infections seen with T-cell deficiencies have been reported in AIDS patients with morphological features of MDS. Patients with CMML and neutrophilic leukocytosis may present with bacterial infections manifested by large collections of pus accumulating within various tissues (pericolic, perinephric, intramuscular). Such infections give rise to very little systemic reaction. Large pus collections and the reduced systemic response may both be related to abnormalities in granulocytic function.

Morphological features of MDS have been reported in patients with AIDS and most likely represent a direct toxic effect of the virus on the bone marrow rather than the evolution of an autonomous myelodysplastic clone. Nevertheless, some authors believe that dysplastic features are the rule rather than the exception. By contrast, and in support of MDS–leukemic transformation, Napoli et al. (1986) reported a case of AIDS-related complex with RAEB-IT who progressed to acute myeloblastic leukemia, suggesting that the dysplastic process in AIDS may be clonal and preleukemic. Also, Sham and Bennett (1992) have described a case of Burkitt cell leukemia with myelodysplasia as a presentation of AIDS.

In support of these unique cases, the feline leukemia virus is capable of producing both MDS and feline AIDS prior to leukemic conversion. Besides the association between HIV, the feline leukemia virus, and AIDS, Baurmann et al. (1992) have documented a case of acute parvovirus B19 infection mimicking MDS. This patient had pancytopenia, splenomegaly, marked dysplastic changes, excess blasts, and spurious red cell precursors.

Clearly, a direct toxic effect from HIV is not the only cause of myelodysplastic changes in AIDS patients. Harris et al. (1990), in evaluating 183 bone marrow, samples from AIDS patients, found that one-third of the marrows yielded specific information. This included opportunistic infection, in particular *Mycobacterium avium-intracellulare* complex, malignancy, and findings consistent with ITP and iron deficiency. In the remaining two-thirds of the bone marrows, the most frequent nonspecific abnormalities were dyserythropoiesis, erythroid hypoplasia, reticuloendothelial iron blockade, granulomas, lymphoid aggregates, plasmacytosis, and histiocytosis. Common peripheral blood findings were anemia, lymphopenia, anisocytosis, rouleaux formation, and the presence of atypical lymphocytes.

The above peripheral blood and bone marrow findings were more pronounced in 16 patients in this series who were receiving zidovudine (azidothymidine, or AZT) treatment.

Therefore, the causes of hematopoietic abnormalities in AIDS are multifactorial. They include severe viral and opportunistic infections, as well as therapy with marrow-toxic drugs.

Autoimmune Disease

Autoimmune disease has been associated with MDS in a number of cases. Mufti et al. (1986) reported a series of 104 patients with MDS; 2 had associated pernicious anemia, 2 had hypothyroidism, and 1 had both conditions. Three patients had seronegative rheumatoid arthritis, but this probably represented a chance associa-

In addition to altered numbers of T cells in MDS, functional abnormalities have been widely reported. Poor lymphoproliferative responses to phytohemagglutinin and concanavalin A have been reported by a number of investigators. Apparently, the poor phytohemagglutinin response could not be corrected in vitro by cimetidine, indomethacin, or isoprinosine, suggesting that the impairment was probably not caused by T-suppressor activity, monocyte suppression, or deficient helper/inducer function, respectively. Furthermore, T-cell cloning efficiency is severely impaired and MDS lymphocytes show increased sensitivity to x-rays. Some investigators have postulated a decreased ability of MDS lymphocytes to mediate DNA repair. This has been supported by a study by Murphy et al. (1984) of the effect of ultraviolet light on lymphocytes from RAEB patients.

In a recent study by Morra et al. (1992), the ability of T lymphocytes to stimulate in vitro growth of circulating erythroid progenitors (BFU-E) and the production of burst-promoting activity (BPA) were significantly reduced in 17 MDS patients. Such studies can supply useful prognostic information concerning the responsiveness of erythropoietic stem cells to recombinant human erythropoietin in vivo.

Finally, Tsukamoto et al. (1993), using X-linked restriction fragment length polymorphisms (RFLP) analysis in six MDS patients, were able to demonstrate a monoclonal pattern of X-inactivation of T lymphocytes and granulocyte fractions. They concluded that the majority of MDS cases arise from a pluripotent stem cell. By contrast, van Kamp et al. (1992), using X-linked RFLP and PCR of the phosphoglycerate kinase gene, showed a nonrandom, unilateral pattern of X-inactivation, compatible with a mixture of clonally (myeloid) and polyclonally (lymphoid) derived cells. They concluded that in some patients the MDS represents a disorder with clonal hematopoiesis restricted to cells of myeloid origin, whereas a random X-inactivation pattern is found in lymphoid cells.

Abnormalities of NK cells

NK cells are usually large, granular lymphocytes that are neither of B-cell nor T-cell lineage. They originate in the bone marrow and characteristically express CD16 and CD56. These cells are unique in that they have the ability to kill certain tumor target cells without requiring the expression of class I or II molecules of the major histocompatibility complex (MHC) by the targets. A small fraction of CD3+ T lymphocytes is also capable of mediating NK activity.

Quantitative evaluation of NK cells has been complex and difficult. Hokland et al. (1986), using HNK-1 (CD57), found reduced numbers of NK cells in 29 of 32 patients with RA and RARS in both peripheral blood and bone marrow. Contrariwise, other investigators using the same monoclonal antibody have found normal percentages of NK cells in peripheral blood of MDS patients.

Impaired NK activity in MDS has been studied by many groups, using the killing of the erythroleukemic cell line K562 as an index of NK activity. All have demonstrated impaired NK activity. Kerndrup and Hokland (1988) extended these studies and not only used K562 cells as a target, but also included two acute T-lymphoblastic leukemia cells, MOLT-4 and 1301, as targets. Again, 11 of 13 patients with RA and RARS showed subnormal NK activity. Further investigation of three patients for antibody-dependent cellular cytotoxicity (ADCC), a property thought to be mediated through NK cells, revealed normal findings.

In contrast, Janowska-Wieczorek et al. (1983) reported markedly reduced levels of ADCC in four patients with RARS.

Nand et al. (1992) treated 20 MDS patients with daily subcutaneous injections of interferon alpha 2a (IFNα2α) with no change in NK activity. They concluded that 1FNα2α was ineffective and toxic. Okabe et al. (1986) found low levels of α-IFN production in 8 of 11 MDS patients in response to stimulation by HeLa-M cells. On the other hand, Soiffer et al. (1992), treating bone marrow transplant patients with recombinant interleukin 2 (IL-2), demonstrated a marked increase in NK cell number but only a minor increase in T-cell number. The implications of these results are under investigation by the authors.

Finally, a study by van Kamp et al. (1992) utilized X-linked RFLP and PCR of the phosphoglycerate kinase gene in 11 female patients with MDS. They showed that Southern blot and PCR analysis were concordant, and that polymorphonuclear cells and monocytes were clonally derived; by contrast, circulating T, B, and NK cells exhibited random X-chromosome inactivation compatible with a polyclonal pattern. This supports the concept that MDS represents a disorder with clonal hematopoiesis restricted to cells of myeloid origin.

Abnormalities of Monocytes

As noted above, both the granulocytic and monocytic series in MDS are clearly derived from an abnormal clone. Such an abnormality has resulted in decreased numbers of both granulocytes and monocytes. Because of this, numerous studies utilizing recombinant growth factors to stimulate granulopoiesis have been undertaken.

In addition, studies have supported monocyte/macrophage dysfunction that accounts for abnormalities in antibody production, suggesting that antigen presentation and secretion of cytokines are impaired. This conclusion is supported by suboptimal phagocytosis of IgG-coated sheep red blood cells by blood and bone marrow monocytes in CMML but not in acute leukemia. On the other hand, evidence for a functional abnormality of monocytes in CMML patients has been minimal, and some studies on phagocytosis of opsonized *Staphylococcus epidermidis* revealed the activity of monocytes to be normal or elevated, with only a few being suboptimal in function. Furthermore, pinocytosis of dextran sulfate was normal in the majority of cases. Also, no difference has been observed between the phagocytosis and intracellular killing of *C. albicans* by peripheral blood and bone marrow monocytes in MDS patients. In conclusion, evaluation of monocytic migration by skin window technique showed normal emigration of blood monocytes to tissue but delayed acquisition of lysosomal enzymes.

Cytochemical abnormalities including decreased levels of nonspecific esterase in peripheral blood monocytes and low levels of myeloperoxidase in peripheral blood and bone marrow monocytes and promonocytes have been reported. DePasquale et al. (1993) documented a case of CMML showing myeloperoxidase-deficient monocytes and normal neutrophils by automated differential cell counting confirmed by cytochemical and immunocytochemical investigations. They attributed the deficiency to a partial maturation arrest of monocytes.

Recently, Ohmori et al. (1992) have studied in vitro colony formation of normal granulocyte-macrophage progenitors. They discovered that monocyte-derived, lipid-containing, huge macrophages developed that suppressed the growth of normal granulocyte-macrophage progenitors. Cell lysates of these macrophages reacted to both monoclonal anti-H subunit ferritin and polyclonal anti-placental ferritin in Western blotting analysis, indicating that the inhibitory activity was predominantly due to acidic isoferritin. On the other hand, similar macrophages obtained from normal bone marrow had granulocyte-macrophage progenitor enhancing activity. These results seem to indicate that these huge macrophages may be responsible for the suppression of granulopoiesis in MDS patients and that such suppression may be mediated by soluble factors, notably H subunit isoferritin.

BIBLIOGRAPHY

Articles

Anderson RW, Volsky DJ, Greenberg B, et al: Lymphocyte abnormalities in preleu-kemia-I. Decreased NK activity, anomalous immunoregulatory cell subsets and deficient EBV receptors. *Leuk Res* 7:389–395, 1983.

Ayanlar-Batuman O, Shevitz J, Traub UC, et al: Lymphocyte interleukin-2 production and responsiveness are altered in patients with primary myelodysplastic syndrome. *Blood* 70:494–500, 1987.

Baumann MA, Milson TJ, Patrick CW, et al: Immunoregulatory abnormalities in myelodysplastic disorders. *Am J Hematol* 22:17–26, 1986.

Baurmann H, Schwarz TF, Oertel J, et al: Acute parvovirus B19 infection mimicking myelodysplastic syndrome of the bone marrow. *Ann Hematol* 64:43–45, 1992.

Bennett JM, Catovsky D, Daniel MT, et al: Criteria for the diagnosis of acute megakaryocytic lineage (M7). *Ann Intern Med* 103:460–462, 1985.

Bettelheim P, Schwarzinger I, Jagear U, et al: Prognostic significance of the immunological marker profile in de novo acute myeloid leukemia (AML). *Blood* 70(Suppl 1):198a, 1987.

Calapso P, Vitarelli E, Crisafulli C, et al: Immunocytochemical detection of mega-karyocytes by endothelial markers: A comparative study. *Pathologica* 84:215–223, 1992.

Candido A, Rossi P, Menichella G, et al: Indicative morphological myelodysplastic alterations of bone marrow in overt AIDS. *Haematologica* 75:327–333, 1990.

Colombat PH, Renoux M, Lamagnere JP, et al: Immunologic indices in myelodys-plastic syndromes. *Cancer* 61:1075–1081, 1988.

Cuneo A, Fagioli F, Pazzi I, et al: Morphologic, immunologic and cytogenetic studies in acute myeloid leukemia following occupational exposure to pesti-cides and organic solvents. *Leuk Res* 16:789–796, 1992.

De-Pasquale A, Ginaldi L, Di Leonardo G, et al: Selective involvement of mono-cytes by acquired myeloperoxidase deficiency in a case of chronic myelomono-cytic leukemia. *Ann Hematol* 66:261–264, 1993.

Economopoulos T, Economidou J, Giannopoulos G, et al: Immune abnormalities in myelodysplastic syndromes. *J Clin Pathol* 38:908–911, 1985.

Fagioli F, Cuneo A, Piva N, et al: Distinct cytogenetic and clinicopathologic features in acute myeloid leukemia after occupational exposure to pesticides and organic solvents. *Cancer* 70:77–85, 1992.

Folks TM: Human immunodeficiency virus in bone marrow. Still more questions than answers (editorial). *Blood* 77:1625–1626, 1991.

Garcia S, Sanz MA, Amigo V, et al: Prognostic factors in chronic myelodysplastic syndromes: A multivariate analysis in 107 cases. *Am J Hematol* 27:163–168, 1988.

Gisslinger H, Gilly B, Woloszczuk W, et al: Thyroid autoimmunity and hypothyroidism during long-term treatment with recombinant interferon-alpha. *Clin Exp Immunol* 90:363–367, 1992.

Groupe Francais de Cytogenetique Hematologique (GFCH): Acute leukemia treated with intensive chemotherapy in patients with a history of previous chemo- and/or radiotherapy: Prognostic significance of karyotype and preceding myelodysplastic syndrome. *Leukemia* 8(1):87–91, 1994.

Guyotat D, Campos L, Thomas X, et al: Myelodysplastic syndromes: A study of surface markers and in vitro growth patterns. *Am J Hematol* 34:26–31, 1990.

Hall AG, Proctor SJ, Saunders PW: Increased platelet associated immunoglobulin in myelodysplastic syndromes. *Br J Haematol* 65:245–246, 1987.

Han K, Lee W, Harris CP, et al: Quantifying chromosome changes and lineage involvement in myelodysplastic syndrome (MDS) using fluorescent in situ hybridization (FISH). *Leukemia* 8(1):81–6, 1994.

Harris CE, Biggs JC, Concannon AJ, et al: Peripheral blood and bone marrow findings in patients with acquired immune deficiency syndrome. *Pathology* 22:206–211, 1990.

Hokland P, Kerndrup G, Griffin JD, et al: Analysis of leukocyte differentiation antigens in blood and bone marrow from preleukemia (refractory anemia) patients using monoclonal antibodies. *Blood* 67:898–902, 1986.

Horny HP, Wehrmann M, Griesser H, et al: Investigation of bone marrow lymphocyte subsets in normal, reactive, and neoplastic states using paraffin-embedded biopsy specimens. *Am J Clin Pathol* 99:142–149, 1993.

Jaeger U, Panzer S, Bartram C, et al: Autoimmune-thrombocytopenia and SLE in a patient with 5q-anomaly and deletion of the c-fms oncogene. *Am J Hematol* 45(1):79–80, 1994.

Janowska-Wieczorek A, Jakobisiak M, Dobsczewska H, et al: Decreased antibody-dependent cellular cytotoxicity in preleukemic syndromes. *Acta Haematol* 69:132–135, 1983.

Janvier G, Junca J, Milla F, et al: Anemia hemolitica autoimmune y sindrome mielodisplasico. *Sangre-Bare* 35:488, 1990.

Kaczmarski RS, Pozniak A, Lakhani A, et al: A pilot study of low-dose recombinant human granulocyte-macrophage colony-stimulating factor in chronic neutropenia. *Br J Haematol* 84:338–340, 1993.

Kawaguchi M, Nehashi Y, Aizawa S, et al: Comparative study of immunocytochemical staining versus Giemsa stain for detecting dysmegakaryopoiesis in myelodysplastic syndromes (MDS). *Eur J Haematol* 44:89–94, 1990.

Kerkhos H, Hermans J, Haak HL, et al: Utility of the FAB classification for myelodysplastic syndromes: Investigation of prognostic factors in 237 cases. *Br J Haematol* 65:73–81, 1987.

Kerndrup G, Hokland P: Natural killer cell-mediated inhibition of bone marrow colony formation (CFU-GM) in refractory anaemia (preleukaemia): Evidence for patient-specific cell populations. *Br J Haematol* 69:457–462, 1988.

Kletter Y, Nagler A: Function of peripheral blood and bone marrow monocytes in preleukemic patients: Normal phagocytosis and intracellular killing of *Candida albicans*. *Acta Haematol* 72:379–383, 1984.

Knox SJ, Greenberg BR, Anderson RW, et al: Studies of T lymphocytes in preleukemic disorders and acute nonlymphocytic leukemia: In vitro radiosensitivity, mitogenic responsiveness, colony formation, and enumeration of lymphocytic subpopulations. *Blood* 61:449–455, 1983.

Martin-Vega C, Vallespi T, Julia A, et al: Anemia hemolitica autoinmune y sindromes mielodisplasicos. *Sangre-Bare* 34:343–345, 1989.

Marulo S, Dallot A, Cavelier-Balloy B, et al: Subcutaneous eosinophilic necrosis associated with refractory anemia with an excess of myeloblasts. *J Am Acad Dermatol* 20:320–323, 1989.

Matutes E, Urbano-Ispizua A, Feliu E, et al: Immunophenotypical features of blast cells in myelodysplastic syndromes. *Blood* 72(Suppl 1):215a, 1988.

Morra L, Moccia F, Ponassi I, et al: In vitro growth of erythroid progenitor cells (BFU-E) and production of burst-promoting activity (BPA) by T lymphocytes in patients with myelodysplastic syndromes. *Biomed Pharmacother* 46:393–399, 1992.

Mostl M, Mucke H, Schinkinger M, et al: Indications for the presence of antibodies cross-reactive with HTLV I/II, but not HIV in patients with myelodysplastic syndrome. *Clin Immunol Immunopathol* 65:75–79, 1992.

Mufti GJ, Figes A, Hamblin TJ, et al: Immunological abnormalities in myelodysplastic syndromes. I. Serum immunoglobulins and autoantibodies. *Br J Haematol* 63:143–147, 1986.

Mullins JI, Chen CS, Hoover EA: Disease-specific and tissue-specific production of unintegrated feline leukaemia virus variant DNA in feline AIDS. *Nature* 319:333–336, 1986.

Murthy PB, Kamada N, Kuramoto A: Defective ultraviolet induced DNA repair in bone marrow cells and peripheral lymphocytes of patients with refractory anemia with excess of blasts. *Jpn J Clin Oncol* 14:87–91, 1984.

Nakayama S, Ishikawa T, Yabe H, et al: Refractory anemia complicated by Behcet's disease—report of three cases. *Rinsho-Ketsueki* 30:530–534, 1989.

Nand S, Ellis T, Messmore H, et al: Phase II trial of recombinant human interferon alpha in myelodysplastic syndromes. *Leukemia* 6:220–223, 1992.

Napoli VM, Stein SF, Spira TJ, et al: Myelodysplasia progressing to acute myeloblastic leukemia in an HTLV-III virus-positive homosexual man with AIDS-related complex. *Am J Clin Pathol* 86:788–791, 1986.

Nylund SJ, Verbeek W, Larramendy ML, et al: Cell lineage involvement in four patients with myelodysplastic syndrome and t(1;7) or trisomy 8 studied by simultaneous immunophenotyping and fluorescence in situ hybridization. *Cancer Genet Cytogenet* 70:120–124, 1993.

Ohmori M, Ueda Y, Masutani H, et al: Myelodysplastic syndrome (MDS)-associated inhibitory activity on haematopoietic progenitor cells: Contribution of monocyte-derived lipid containing macrophages. *Br J Haematol* 81:67–72, 1992.

Okabe M, Minagawa T, Nakane A, et al: Impaired α-interferon production and natural killer activity in blood mononuclear cells in myelodysplastic syndromes. *Scand J Haematol* 37:111–117, 1986.

Orazi A, Cattoretti G, Soligo D, et al: Therapy-related myelodysplastic syndromes:

FAB classification, bone marrow histology, and immunohistology in the prognostic assessment. *Leukemia* 7:838–847, 1993.

Porzsolt F, Heimpel H: Impaired T-cell and NK-cell function in patients with preleukemia. *Blut* 45:243–248, 1982.

Ramakrishna R, Chaudhuri K, Sturgess A, et al: Haematological manifestations of primary Sjogren's syndrome: A clinicopathological study. *Q J Med* 83:547–554, 1993.

Reading CL, Estey EH, Huk YO, et al: Expression of unusual immunophenotype combinations in acute myelogenous leukemia. *Blood* 81:3083–3090, 1993.

Reboli AC, Reilly RF, Jacobson RJ: Aspergillus myositis in a patient with a myelodysplastic syndrome. *Mycopathologia* 97:117–119, 1987.

Rockley PF, Bergfeld WF, Tomecki KJ, et al: Myelodysplastic syndrome and transient acantholytic dermatosis. *Cleve Clin J Med* 57:575–577, 1990.

San Miguel JF, Gonzalez M, Canizo MC, et al: The nature of blast cells in myelodysplastic syndromes evolving to acute leukaemia. *Blut* 52:357–361, 1986.

Sanz C, Cervantes F, Pereira A, et al: Anemia hemolitica autoinmune Coombs positiva como manifestacion in cial destacoda de los sindromes mielodisplasicos. *Sangre-Bare* 35:329, 1990.

Shneider DR, Picker LJ: Myelodysplasia in the acquired immune deficiency syndrome. *Am J Clin Pathol* 84:144–152, 1985.

Seitanides B, Antonopoulou A, Karabelis A: Immunological abnormalities in myelodysplastic syndrome. *J Clin Pathol* 41:922–923, 1988.

Seo IS, Li-Cy Yam LT: Myelodysplastic syndrome: Diagnostic implications of cytochemical and immunocytochemical studies. *Mayo Clin Proc* 68:47–53, 1993.

Seyfried H, Walewska I: Analysis of immune response to red blood cell antigens in multitransfused patients with different diseases. *Mater Med Pol* 22:21–25, 1990.

Sham RL, Bennett JM: Burkitt cell leukemia with myelodysplasia as a presentation of HIV infection. *Hematol Pathol* 6:95–98, 1992.

Shitara T, Yugami S, Sotomatu M, et al: Invasive aspergillosis in leukemic children. *Pediatr Hematol Oncol* 10:169–174, 1993.

Soiffer RJ, Murray C, Cochran K, et al: Clinical and immunologic effects of prolonged infusion of low dose recombinant interleukin-2 after autologous and T-cell-depleted allogeneic bone marrow transplantation. *Blood* 79:517–526, 1992.

Solal-Celigny P, Desaint B, Herrera A, et al: Chronic myelomonocytic leukemia according to FAB classification: Analysis of 35 cases. *Blood* 63:634–638, 1984.

Sonnevelu P, Van-Dongen JJ, Hagemeijer A, et al: High expression of the multidrug resistance P-glycoprotein in high-risk myelodysplasia is associated with immature phenotype. *Leukemia* 7:963–969, 1993.

Stark AN, Scott CS, Roberts BE: Coexistent lymphoid or plasma cell neoplasms. *Br J Haematol* 65:376–377, 1987.

Tallman MS, McGuffin RW, Higano CS, et al: Bone marrow transplantation in a patient with myelodysplasia associated with diffuse eosinophilic fascitis. *Am J Hematol* 24:93–99, 1987.

Tanaka K, Nakamura E, Naitoh K, et al: Relapsing polychondritis in a patient with myelodysplastic syndrome. *Rinsho-Ketsueki* 31:1851–1855, 1990.

Teerenhovi L, Lintula R: Natural course of myelodysplastic syndrome—Helsinki experience. *Scand J Haematol* 45(Suppl):102–106, 1986.

Thiele J, Quitman H, Wagner S, et al: Dysmegakaryopoiesis in myelodysplastic syndromes (MDS): An immunomorphometric study of bone marrow trephine biopsy specimens. *J Clin Pathol* 44:300–305, 1991.

Tsukamoto N, Morita K, Maehara T, et al: Clonality in myelodysplastic syndromes: Demonstration of pluriopotent stem cell origin using X-linked restriction fragment length polymorphisms. *Br J Haematol* 83:589–594, 1993.

Van Furth R, van Zwet TL: Cytochemical, functional, and proliferative characteristics of promonocytes and monocytes from patients with monocytic leukemia. *Blood* 62:298–304, 1983.

Van-Kamp H, Fibbe WE, Jansen RP, et al: Clonal involvement of granulocytes and monocytes, but not T and B lymphocytes and natural killer cells in patients with myelodysplasia: Analysis by X-linked restriction fragment length polymorphisms and polymerase chain reaction of the phosphoglycerate kinase gene. *Blood* 80:1774–1780, 1992.

Visani G, Tosi P, Finelli C, et al: Effect of in vivo treatment with rh GM-CSF on in vitro growth of haematopoietic progenitors in patients with myelodysplastic syndrome. *Haemotologica* 77:142–145, 1992.

Walker RE, Parker RI, Kovacs JA, et al: Anemia and erythropoiesis in patients with the acquired immunodeficiency syndrome (AIDS) and Kaposi's sarcoma treated with zidovudine. *Ann Intern Med* 108:372–376, 1988.

Warren AJ, Hegde UM, Nathwani A, et al: Systemic vasculitis and myelodysplasia. *Br J Haematol* 75:627–629, 1990.

Williamson PJ, Oscier DG, Mufti JM, et al: Pyogenic abscesses in the myelodysplastic syndrome. *Br Med J* 299:375–376, 1989.

Zwiezina H, Sepp N, Ringler E, et al: Delayed maturation of skin window macrophages in myelodysplastic syndromes. *Leuk Res* 13:433–435, 1989.

Review Articles

Hamblin TJ: Immunologic abnormalities in myelodysplastic syndromes. In Mufti GJ, Galton DAG (eds): *The Myelodysplastic Syndromes.* New-York, Churchill Livingstone, 1992, pp 97–114.

Ho PJ, Gibson J, Vincent P, et al: The myelodysplastic syndromes: Diagnostic criteria and laboratory evaluation. *Pathology* 25:297–304, 1993.

Koeller U, Krieger O, Haas OA, et al: Immunological phenotyping of blood and bone marrow cells from patients with myelodysplastic syndromes. In Schmalzl F, Mufti GJ (eds): *Myelodysplastic Syndromes.* New York, Springer-Verlag, 1992, pp 60–66.

Kouides PA, Bennett JM: Morphology and classification of myelodysplastic syndromes. *Hematol Oncol Clin North Am* 6:485–499, 1992.

CHAPTER **7**

Cytogenetics

INTRODUCTION

Since the MDSs represent clonal abnormalities of hematopoietic stem cells that may undergo leukemic proliferation, it is not surprising that approximately 50% of patients with primary MDSs have abnormal karyotypes. In secondary or therapy-related MDS (t-MDS), the incidence of chromosomal abnormalities has been found to be even higher than in primary MDS. In the evaluation of combined data from five large series, Bloomfield (1986) determined an incidence of up to 86% karyotypic abnormalities in t-MDS patients.

Primary MDS may present with either single or multiple chromosomal abnormalities. Initially, the karyotype may demonstrate a single abnormality, but additional changes may occur during the course of the disease, especially with leukemic evolution. Simple chromosome changes are usually observed in the less aggressive forms of primary MDS, i.e., RA and RARS, whereas RAEB and RAEB-T are often characterized by complex karyotypes with multiple abnormalities. They constitute a single numerical change, a structural abnormality involving only one chromosome, or a translocation involving two or more chromosomes. In a small number of cases, two or more unrelated clones with simple chromosomal abnormalities may be observed (5%). Single chromosomal changes observed in primary MDS are depicted in Table 7.1. Complex karyotypes usually involve abnormalities of chromosomes 5 and/or 7.

In contrast to primary MDSs, secondary or t-MDSs tend to show multiple chromosome changes at diagnosis. However, single chromosome changes includ-

Table 7.1   Single-Chromosome Changes in Primary MDS

-7
$+8$
-5 or del(5)(q13-q33) and unbalanced translocations involving 5q
del(7q)
del(11q)-q14 is always involved in either interstitial or terminal deletions
del(12)(p11p13)
del(13q)-q14 is always involved in interstitial deletions of variable size
del(20)(q11q13)
t(1;3)(p36;q21)
t(2;11)(p21;q23)
t(6;9)(p23;q34) very rare
t(11;21)(q24;q11.2)
i(17q) idic(X)(q13)

Source: Sandberg AA, Wullich B: Myelodysplastic syndromes: Cytogenetic anomalies and their clinical significance. In Schmalzl F, Mufti (eds): *Myelodysplastic Syndromes*. New York, Churchill Livingstone, 1992, pp 165–177 (with modification).

ing del(5q) or -5 and del(7q) or -7 have been described. In addition, del(12p) has been demonstrated as a single abnormality. The majority of karyotypic changes in cases with t-MDS involve abnormalities of chromosomes 5 and/or 7, either alone or in combination. Le Beau et al. (1993), in evaluating 63 patients with t-MDS and AML, showed that 98% of patients with t-MDS showed a clonal chromosomal abnormality, and 94% had abnormalities of chromosomes 5 and/or 7. Additional chromosomes frequently involved in multiple aberrations were chromosome 3[del(3p),inv(3)] and chromosome 17 (deletions, translocations involving 17p, and, less frequently, 17q or monosomy). Chromosome changes in t-MDS demonstrate some extraordinary aspects: The karyotype may show genetic instability with minor variations from cell to cell or karyotypic evolution, resulting in multiple clones and monoclonal, abnormal cells with related abnormalities.

In contrast to primary MDS, the presence of complex karyotypes in secondary or t-MDSs is often associated with an inability to classify the disorder into one of the FAB subtypes. This is due to the fact that the majority of t-MDSs demonstrate trilineage features involving different cell lines. The presence of dicentrics and rings can be observed in t-MDS cases and may be related to prior exposure to cytotoxic therapy. Common chromosome changes observed in t-MDS are depicted in Table 7.2.

SPECIFIC CHROMOSOMAL ENTITIES

Abnormalities of Chromosome 5

Van den Berghe et al. described the first case of the 5q− syndrome in 1974. This syndrome has been extensively studied and confirmed, not only for its morphological features—macrocytic anemia, normal or high platelet counts, non-lobulated micromegakaryocytes, and hypoplastic erythroid series— but also for its clinical course, in which evolution to acute leukemia is most uncommon. The

Table 7.2   Common Chromosome Changes in Therapy-Related MDS

Single chromosome changes
+8
del(5q)
del(7q)
−5
−7
del(12p)
del(11q)
del(20q)
del(13q)
t(2;11)(p21;q23)
t(6,9)(p23;q34)
der(1;7)(q10;p10)
Multiple chromosome changes (any of the above plus)
+21
del(3p) or t(3p)
del(17p) or t(17p), del(17q) or t(17q), −17
6p(del or t)

Source: Sandberg AA, Wullich B: Myelodysplastic syndromes: Cytogenetic anomalies and their clinical significance. In Schmalzl F, Mufti (eds): *Myelodysplastic Syndromes.* New York, Churchill Livingstone, 1992, pp 165–177 (with modification).

disorder is a distinct hematological abnormality occurring primarily in elderly women. The typical del(5q) chromosome change occurs in a multipotential stem cell and is usually present at the time the hematological abnormalities of the disorder are identified. However, cases can occur in which only a normal karyotype is seen at diagnosis, with detection of the typical del(5q) later in the course of RA. The bone marrow resembles several FAB subtypes of MDS (RA, RARS, RAEB), with the presence of monolobated micromegakaryocytes as a constant feature.

Even though the breakpoints and the extent of the deletions of the 5q are variable, the character of the deletions in the del(5q) syndrome, as well as of those in t-MDS/t-AML and MDS/AML de novo, appears to be relatively similar, with a proximal breakpoint frequently at band q13–q15 and a distal breakpoint within region q3 at bands q31-35. Evaluation of t-MDS/t-AML, MDS, AML de novo, and RA by Le Beau et al. (1993) revealed deletion of a region called the critical region consisting of band 5q31, which occurs in all patients (Fig. 7.1). This critical region has recently been narrowed to a small segment (approximately 2.8 megabases) of 5q31 containing the *EGR1* gene.

Although the critical region is involved in all patients in the del(5q) anomaly, deletions have sometimes been interpreted as terminal and sometimes as interstitial, with all bands between 5q11 and 5q35 implicated as breakpoints. The majority of reports have concluded that the deletion is interstitial, and the breakpoints most frequently reported are 5q21–14 (proximal molecular breakpoint) and q31–q33 (distal breakpoint). Furthermore, molecular studies and fluorescence in situ hybridization analysis have demonstrated that the deletions are interstitial. A minimal common deleted segment on 5q has been identified at 5q31 in various malignant disorders associated with del(5q). Many types of interstitial deletions

CRITICAL REGION ON CHROMOSOME 5

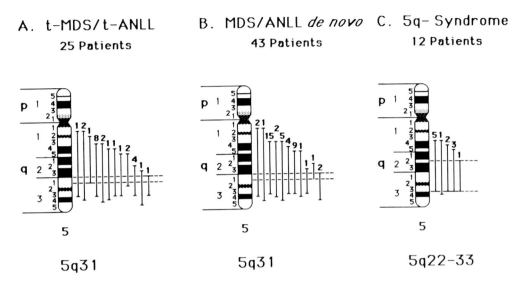

A. t-MDS/t-ANLL

25 Patients

B. MDS/ANLL *de novo*

43 Patients

C. 5q- Syndrome

12 Patients

5q31

5q31

5q22-33

Figure 7.1 Diagram of the banding pattern of chromosome 5, illustrating the chromosomal breakpoints and deletions in patients with t-MDS/t-AML, MDS/AML de novo, and the 5q− syndrome. Each vertical bar represents the region that was deleted; the numbers above the lines indicate the number of patients with this deletion. The dashed horizontal lines indicate the critical region, i.e., the smallest overlapping region that was deleted in each of the patients. (Courtesy of Michelle M. LeBeau).

have been recognized; however, the three most common ones—del(5)(q13q33), del(5)(q14q33), and del(5)(q15q33)—account for approximately 85%.

There are a number of relevant candidate genes within or adjacent to the critical region of 5q whose function suggests a possible role in the pathogenesis of myeloid disorders. These candidate genes encode a variety of growth factors and growth factor receptors (Fig. 7.2). Five of these genes encode hematopoietic growth factors, three of which are colony-stimulating factors (CSFs), a family of glycoprotein growth factors that are required for growth and maturation of myeloid progenitor cells in vivo.

By in situ chromosomal hybridization and the analysis of somatic hybrids, interleukin 3 (IL-3, 5q31), granulocyte, macrophage CSF-2/GM-CSF, 5q31, IL-4 (5q31), IL-5 (5q31), IL-9 (5q31), and FMS (5q33) genes have been localized to chromosome 5. Recently, Le Beau et al. (1993) have further characterized the distal 5q region or the smallest commonly deleted region of chromosome 5 in malignant myeloid disease. This region contains a number of genes encoding hematopoietic growth factors (CSF-2, IL-3, IL-4, IL-5, and IL-9), hormone receptors, and proteins involved in signal transduction or transcriptional regulation and has been localized to 5q31.1. By molecular studies, the critical region was shown to be approximately 2.8 megabases in length and contains the *EGR*1 gene. The genes encoding IL-3, GM-CSF, IL-4, IL-5, and IL-9 are proximal to this region and are not deleted in all patients.

Additional genes mapped to the distal long arm of chromosome 5 include

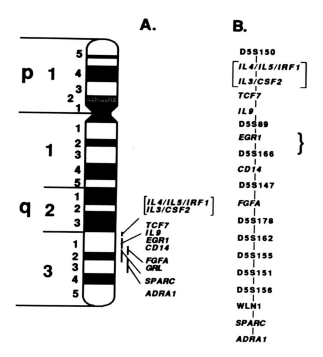

Figure 7.2 Schematic diagram of the banding pattern of chromosome 5 illustrating the chromosomal localization and order of the IL-4/IL-5/IRF-1, IL-3/CSF2, TCF7, IL-9, EGR1, CD14, FGFA, GRL, SPARC, and ADRA1 genes determined by FISH **(a)** and the physical order of cosmid and phage clones and genes and the relationship of loci on 5q to the critical region of 5q31 (brace) **(b).** Brackets identify probes for which the order is unknown. (From M.M. LeBeau. Proc. Natl. Acad. Sci USA 90:5486, 1993.)

genes encoding the myeloid-specific antigen, CD14, the platelet-derived growth factor receptor (PDGFR), the β_2-adrenergic and α_1-adrenergic receptors (ADRA$_1$), glucocorticoid receptor, and endothelial cell growth factor (ECGF). These genes are excluded from the commonly deleted segment. The *EGR1* gene within the critical region is unique in that it encodes a 533 amino acid protein that contains three DNA-binding zinc fingers, a motif that is characteristic of proteins capable of binding to DNA and regulating gene expression. The *EGR1* gene is required for differentiation of monocytic cells and plays an important role in hematopoiesis. Although the *EGR1* gene is a candidate tumor suppressor gene in myeloid leukemogenesis, mutations of *EGR1* have not yet been identified in leukemias characterized by a del(5q).

From the above findings, the properties of the *EGR1* gene; its location within the critical region which is deleted in all patients with t-MDS/t-AML, MDS, AML de novo, or RA with deletion of 5q; and its encoded protein suggest that this gene is a more suitable candidate for playing a role in the malignant transformation of myeloid cells with a del(5q) than are the genes that encode growth factors or receptors.

The development of a cytogenetic map of 5q by Le Beau et al. (1993), together with molecular characterization of the critical region, will facilitate the identification of a putative tumor suppressor gene.

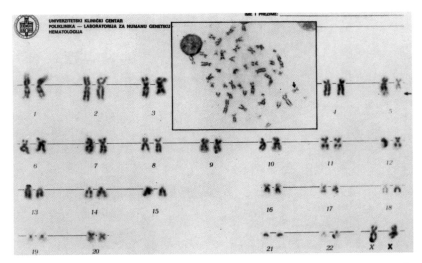

Figure 7.3a G-banded karyotype and metaphase. Arrows indicate interstitial deletion 5q. (From Novak A, Jankovic G, Rolovic Z: Two karyotypically unrelated clones with t(5;17) and deletion of 5q in myelodysplastic syndrome. *Cancer Genet Cytogenet* 62:100–102, 1992. Reprinted with permission.)

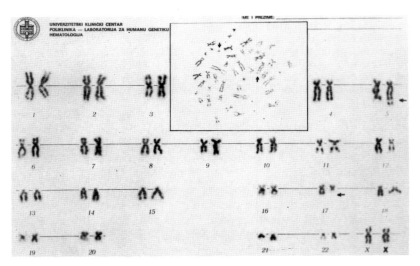

Figure 7.3b Karyotype and metaphse of a G-banded cell showing t(5;17). Arrows indicate abnormal chromosomes 5 and 17. (From Novak A, Jankovic G, Rolovic Z: Two karyotypically unrelated clones with t(5;17) and deletion of 5q in myelodysplastic syndrome. *Cancer Genet Cytogenet* 62:100–102, 1992. Reprinted with permission.)

The clinical course of patients with del(5q) as the sole abnormality (5q− syndrome) is often mild compared to that of patients with secondary or t-MDS, which is usually accompanied by additional aberrations. This strongly supports the concept that the deletion of the critical region (5q31.1) represents only one piece in the complex puzzle of the pathogenesis and disease we designate *leukemogenesis* and *leukemia*, respectively.

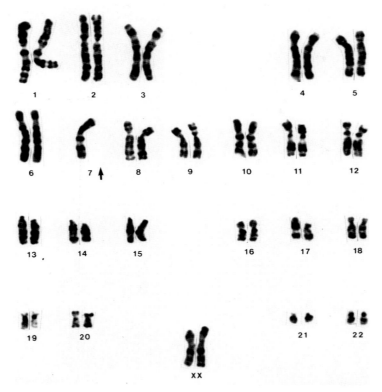

Figure 7.4 Trypsin-Giemsa banded karyotype from a bone marrow aspirate of a patient who has RAEB, illustrating monosomy 7 in a metaphase cell. The karyotype is 45,XX,−7 (arrow). (Courtesy of Ashok K. Srivastava.)

Karyotypes from a patient with a bone marrow mosaicism with a 5q− syndrome is shown in Fig. 7.3. The different chromosomal abnormalities in other metaphases appear to support the multistep theory of pathogenesis in MDS.

Monosomy 7 and Deletions of 7q

Monosomy 7 is one of the most common anomalies in both primary and secondary MDS (t-MDS), as well as in AML and MPD, including juvenile chronic myeloid leukemia. Patients with monosomy 7 have a short survival and a predisposition to develop severe infections. In children, monosomy 7 occurs as a distinct multipotential stem cell disorder associated with recurring infections, abnormal neutrophil chemotaxis, and bacterial killing (familial monosomy 7 syndrome) that is rapidly transformed into overt leukemia. The familial predisposition and age of onset suggest that familial monosomy 7 may show similarities to various solid tumors in children in whom expression of recessive genes has been implicated, such as retinoblastoma. Besides familial monosomy 7, Fanconi's anemia and Down's syndrome demonstrate a monosomy 7 once the disorder evolves to AML or MDS. A trypsin-Giemsa banded karyotype from a patient with RAEB showing monosomy 7 is depicted in Fig. 7.4.

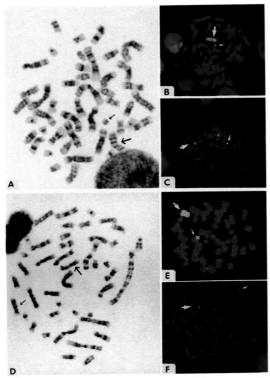

Figure 7.5 Identification of marker chromosomes in two MDS patients **(a–c)** and **(d–f)** by G-banding (A,D) and FISH utilizing either a DNA library probe (pBS7 from Dr. Joe Gray) that hybridizes to the entire length of chromosome 7 **(b,e)** or an alpha-satellite DNA probe that hybridizes specifically to the centromere of chromosome 7 **(c,f)**. Large arrows: normal chromosomes 7; small arrows: marker chromosomes. The mar in patient **(a–c)** is a tiny ring chromosome derived from chromosome 7; the mar was lost in 4/10 metaphases. In patient **(d–f),** one of the two markers contains the chromosome 7p− arm and centromere; this marker was lost in 5/37 metaphases. (From Zhao L, van-Oort J, Cork A, et al: Comparison between interphase and metaphase cytogenetics in detecting chromosome 7 defects in hematological neoplasias. *Am J Hematol* 43:205–211, 1993. Reprinted with permission.)

Recently, there has been a number of studies using fluorescent in situ hybridization (FISH) in monosomy 7 patients. Zhao et al. (1993), comparing FISH with classical cytogenetic techniques, showed that metaphase FISH detected chromosome 7 aberrant sequences undetectable by G-banding. Kadam et al. (1993), also utilizing FISH, discovered masked monosomy 7 in AML. Finally, some investigators have combined immunophenotyping and FISH to investigate monosomy 7–associated disorders. They were able to determine lineage involvement of the monosomic clone which was found in virtually all myelomonocytic and erythroid cells. A G-banding karyotype and FISH of monosomy 7 are shown in two MDS patients in Fig. 7.5. In addition to its usefulness in monosomy 7, FISH has been found to be advantageous in the verification of recurring chromosomal abnormalities. Chen et al. (1993) identified single-cell trisomy in patients with +8, +12, +15, +18, +20 and +21 by classical cytogenetics and confirmed the clonality of these nonrandom abnormalities by the use of FISH. Besides FISH, Abrahamson et al.

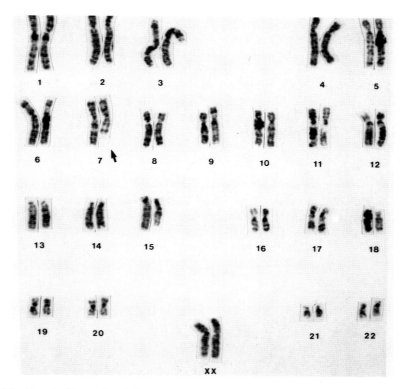

Figure 7.6 Trypsin-Giemsa banded metaphase cell from a bone marrow aspirate of a patient with RAEB-IT illustrating an interstitial deletion in the long arm of chromosome 7 (arrow). The karyotype is 46,XX,del(7)(q21q34). (Courtesy of Ashok K. Srivastava.)

(1993) have used classical cytogenetics and RFLP to detect loss of chromosome 7 in 72 patients with a clonal myeloid malignancy. There were nine cases in which loss of chromosome 7 was detected by both techniques, but in seven loss was detected by only one method, demonstrating the complementary nature of these two techniques.

The deletions of 7q, similar to those of del(5q), are variable, extending from q11 to q36, and are mostly interstitial. Analysis of 38 patients with MDS/AML de novo or t-MDS/t-AML who had a del(7q) suggests that there may be two different critical regions on 7q, namely, 7q22–7q31 and 7q32–7q34 (M. Thangavelu and M.M. Le Beau, unpublished observations). The critical region, by studies at the molecular level, appears to be at 7q22–7q31.2, but the identity of relevant genes on this chromosome is currently unknown. However, *MET*, a proto-oncogene deleted in leukemia cells with a del(7q), has been mapped to 7q31. Furthermore, the gene encoding p glycoprotein, a protein associated with multidrug resistance, and erythropoietin have been localized to 7q21–7q22. Whether hemizygosity for these genes plays a role in malignant transformation is under investigation. A trypsin-Giemsa banded metaphase cell from a patient with RAEB-IT depicting an interstitial deletion in the long arm of chromosome 7 is shown in Fig. 7.6.

Besides monosomy 7 and deletions of 7q, rare cases of centromeric fusion in

7p/1q translocation associated with a secondary MDS have been reported. The karyotype and FISH using ONCOR's chromosome 7-specific (D7Z1) or chromosome 1(D1Z5)-specific centromeric α-satellite DNA probes were employed to characterize the bone marrow karyotype (Fig. 7.7). Initially, the bone marrow karyotype was considered to be 46,XY,−7,+der(1)t(1;7)(p11;p11). However, FISH suggested the presence of both chromosome 1 and chromosome 7 centromeres in the rearranged chromosome. Thus, the correct karyotype should be written as 46,XY,−7,+der(1;7)(q10;p10).

Deletion of 20q

Deletion of the long arm of chromosome 20 may be found in approximately 5% of all MDS patients. However, it is found less often in patients with RA than in other FAB subgroups. Also, the del(20q) is well known in the MPDs—especially in polycythemia vera, where it is the most common aberration occurring in ^{32}P-treated and untreated patients. Davis et al. (1984), in a review of the literature on del(20q) cases, found that 40% of patients had polycythemia vera, 30% had preleukemia, 20%

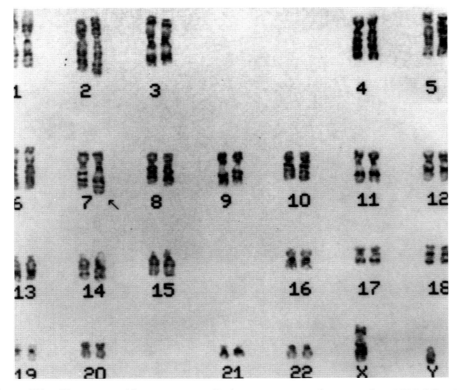

Figure 7.7a Karyogram of bone marrow cells from a patient with a secondary MDS following chemotherapy and radiation therapy showing a 7p/1q translocation chromosome replacing one chromosome 7 (arrow). (From Hoo JJ, Szego K, Jones B: Confirmation of centromeric fusion in 7p/1q translocation associated with myelodysplastic syndrome. *Cancer Genet Cytogenet* 64:187, 1992. Reprinted with permission.)

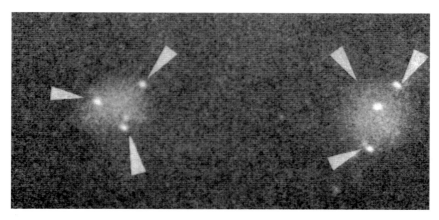

Figure 7.7b   Three signals in both interphase nuclei after hybridization with a chromosome 1-specific centromeric α-satellite probe (D1Z5). (From Hoo JJ, Szego K, Jones B: Confirmation of centromeric fusion in 7p/1q translocation associated with myelodysplastic syndrome. *Cancer Genet Cytogenet* 64:187, 1992. Reprinted with permission.)

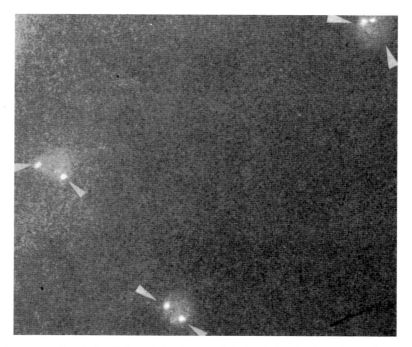

Figure 7.7c   Two signals in all three interphase nuclei after hybridization with a chromosome 7-specific centromeric α-satellite probe (D7Z1). (From Hoo JJ, Szego K, Jones B: Confirmation of centromeric fusion in 7p/1q translocation associated with myelodysplastic syndrome. *Cancer Genet Cytogenet* 64:188, 1992. Reprinted with permission.)

had some kind of myeloproliferative disorder, and 10% had AML. Rare cases have been observed in nonmyeloid neoplasms. Recently, Menke et al. (1992) reported cases of refractory thrombocytopenia, a myelodysplastic syndrome that may mimic immune thrombocytopenic purpura. All patients had oval macrocytes in the peripheral blood and abnormal megakaryocytes in the bone marrow, lacked platelet antibodies, and did not have splenomegaly. The most common clonal chromosomal abnormalities involved chromosomes 3, 5, 8, or 20.

Molecular studies have shown that deletions of 20q are interstitial rather than terminal, as described in previous reports. The most common deletion results from breakpoints at q11.2 and q13.3 [del(20) (q11.2q13.3]. Le Beau et al. (1985) have shown that the *SRC* locus, at 20q11.2 was consistently preserved in leukemia cells with the del(20q). Besides the *SRC* locus, a second oncogene, hemopoietic cell kinase (HCK), whose protein product has tyrosine-kinase activity, has been localized to the long arm of chromosome 20 at bands q11–q12. Since HCK is expressed only by hematopoietic cells and has proximity to one of the breakpoints (q11) of the deletions of 20q, a role for this oncogene in leukemogenesis requires careful study. Nevertheless, a still unidentified gene on the long arm of chromosome 20 may be the pertinent gene whose loss results in malignant transformation.

Deletions of 13q

Even though deletions of 13q are most common in the MPDs, accounting for 10% of cytogenetically abnormal cases of polycythemia vera and myelofibrosis, this abnormality is also observed in MDS and AML. Apparently, there is no predilection for a specific FAB subgroup. The deletions are sometimes reported as terminal and sometimes as interstitial; although the deletion is variable, band 13q14 is consistently lost. Deletion of this band has been seen in a variety of other malignancies, most conspicuously retinoblastoma. Even though the retinoblastoma gene in band 13q14 has been cloned and characterized, it is not known whether the same gene is involved in leukemogenesis.

Trisomy 8

Although trisomy 8 is the single most frequently acquired aberration in AML, in MDS it constitutes the second most common anomaly after del(5q). Trisomy 8 may be seen alone or together with other anomalies and shows no marked frequency differences among FAB subgroups. Even though trisomy is commonly encountered in primary MDS, it seems to be more common in secondary disease (t-MDS). The biological role of trisomy 8 in MDS is not known; however, a gain of a whole chromosome results in gene amplification. Diaz et al. (1985) did not observe gross DNA sequence rearrangements close to or within two oncogenes, *MYC* and *MOS*, located on chromosome 8, in 15 of 16 patients with myeloid diseases. Nevertheless, the presence of subtle mutations, i.e., point mutations and expression of these genes in myeloid leukemia cells, have not yet been examined. Oncogenes recently mapped to chromosome 8 (*LYN* and *PVT*1) have not been investigated in malignant cells with trisomy 8. A FISH with the 8 centromere probe utilized on bone marrow cells from a patient with RAEB-IT is shown in Fig. 7.8.

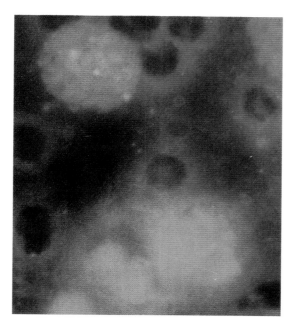

Figure 7.8   Patient with RAEB-IT showing use of the 8 centromere probe by the FISH technique. Note the cell in the upper left corner demonstrating three signals confirming the presence of trisomy 8. (From Han K, Lee W, Harris CP, et al: Quantifying chromosome changes and lineage involvement in myelodysplastic syndrome [MDS] using fluorescent *in situ* hybridization [FISH]. *Leukemia* 8:81–86, 1994. Reprinted with permission.)

Deletion of 11q

Approximately 7% of karyotypic abnormalities in primary MDSs show a deletion of part of chromosome 11q. The deletions usually occur in patients with RARS. Breakpoints are commonly observed in q13 and q23. The commonly deleted segment involves 11q22.3–q23.1. The *MLL* gene at 11q23, which is involved in more than 20 recurring translocations in AML and ALL, is not implicated in these deletions (*MLL* is distal to the commonly deleted segment). A trypsin-Giemsa banded metaphase from a bone marrow aspirate from an RARS patient is shown in Fig. 7.9.

Deletion of 12p

In 5% of cases with primary MDSs, a 12p karyotypic abnormality is observed. This abnormality occurs commonly in chronic myelomonocytic leukemia. *c-K-RAS* 2 is localized at 12p12 to 12pter; however, involvement of this gene in the del(12p) has not yet been demonstrated.

i(17q)

This isochromosome, which is one of the frequent additional aberrations that occur in CML in blast crisis, is also found in 2% of MDS cases. The numbers are

Table 7.3   Recurrent Aberrations

Aberrations Common to MDSs and AML	Aberrations Common to MDSs and MPDs
t(1;3)(p36;q21)	dup (1q)
t(2;11)(p21;q23)	i(17q)
t(3;5)(q25;q34)	idic(X)(q13)
inv(3)(q21q26)/t(3;3)(q21;q26)	−7/del(7q) or −5/del(5q)
+4	+8
+11	inv(3)(q21q26)/t(3;3)(q21;q26)
−Y	del(13q)
−7/del(7q) or −5/del(5q)	der(1;7)(q10;p10)

Source: Sandberg AA, Wullich B: Myelodysplastic syndromes: Cytogenetic anomalies and their clinical significance. In Schmalzl F, Mufti GJ (eds): *Myelodysplastic Syndromes*. New York, Churchill Livingstone, 1992, pp 165–177 (with modification).
Abbreviations: t = translocation; inv = inversion; i = isochromosome.

investigations, irrespective of FAB status, have begun to modify this conclusion by demonstrating that the increased risk is primarily associated with clones that have multiple chromosomal abnormalities or have a single abnormality involving loss of chromosome 7 or 7q. Recent studies by Maschek et al. (1993) evaluating 352 patients with primary MDS have shown that karyotypic abnormalities involving particularly chromosome 7 seem to be associated with hypoplastic MDS. Median survival of the hypoplastic group (42 patients) was intermediate between that of the normoplastic and the hyperplastic group. Although RA patients with 5q− as the only abnormality have a good long-term prognosis, it is not yet clear whether other single chromosome abnormalities that occur nonrandomly in MDSs, such as +8, i(17q), del(20), and balanced translocations, have independent prognostic significance.

There is a general consensus that the appearance of an abnormal chromosomal clone in a MDS patient with a previously normal karyotype, or the emergence of additional changes in a previously abnormal clone, usually portends accelerated disease and a poor outcome.

Although the prognostic value of cytogenetic analysis has previously been demonstrated in MDS, the karyotype has not been included in previously published scoring systems, i.e., Bournemouth and Sanz's scores. Recently, Morel et al. (1993) studied 408 cases of de novo MDS and classified them into 10 groups. Karyotypes were considered complex when at least three chromosomes were rearranged. Complex karyotypes included all patients with del(5q) and other rearrangements, −7 or del(7q) and other rearrangements, and miscellaneous complex rearrangements. Bone marrow blasts, circulating blasts, white blood cell count, neutrophil count, platelet count, hemoglobin, age, sex, FAB classification, and Bournemouth and Sanz's scores had strong prognostic value. Cytogenetic analysis also showed strong predictive ability. The authors developed a new three-variable scoring system (Lille score) which included karyotype, bone marrow blasts, and platelets. The Lille score subdivided risk groups according to Bournemouth and Sanz's scores into further groups of different prognosis.

Suciu et al. (1990), in evaluating 120 patients with de novo MDS, determined that transformation to acute leukemia was observed in 25% of patients with a normal karyotype, 41% of patients with single anomalies, and 50% of patients with multiple anomalies. The incidence of leukemic transformation was significantly higher in patients with multiple abnormalities. Also, no chromosomal abnormality was especially associated with any group of the FAB classification. Finally, the authors concluded that the FAB classification and chromosomal anomalies were of independent prognostic significance.

Toyama et al. (1993) reported on 401 patients with MDS in a multicentric study in Japan in which they correlated chromosomal findings, leukemic transformation, and prognosis. These findings supported those of Morel et al. and Sucui et al. They observed that the time lapse between MDS diagnosis and development of the leukemic phase and death was significantly shorter in patients with complex karyotypic aberrations than in those without such changes.

In general, patients with t-MDS tend to have more frequent and more massive cytogenetic changes than those with primary MDS. Early identification of these and other subsets with an unfavorable prognosis by karyotypic analysis may help to pinpoint those patients who are most likely to benefit from a more aggressive therapeutic approach.

Recently, Pederson (1992) reported on two patients with der(1;7) (q10;p10), which has been associated with MDS and AML, and reviewed the literature. Thirty-six of 73 patients had a history of exposure to chemotherapy or radiotherapy. Alkylating agents were used in 29 patients. The prognosis was poor, with a median survival of only 11 months.

Children seem to have the more aggressive types of MDS. Nair et al. (1992), in evaluating 16 children with MDS, revealed that 7, 6, and 3 were classified as having RAEB, RAEB-IT, and CMML, respectively. Cytogenetic analysis performed in 7 of the 16 patients showed karyotypic abnormalities involving chromosomes 7, 8, and 17. Mean duration of survival was only 5.5, months and aggressive chemotherapy was employed. The predominance of aggressive types of MDS in children, and their good but brief response to aggressive chemotherapy, suggest the need for early bone marrow transplantation in these cases.

Finally, Sullivan et al. (1992), in a survey of 62 MDS patients over a 2-year period, used cytogenetics, CFU-GM colony growth, and assessment of circulating CD34+ cells. They determined that the presence of circulating CD34+ cells was significantly associated with both progression to AML and poor survival, and was found to be a better prognostic indicator than cytogenetic analysis or CFU-GM colony growth. Nevertheless, in more recent series, cytogenetics has been shown to be the strongest independent predictor of the response to treatment.

BIBLIOGRAPHY

Articles

Abrahamsosn GM, Rack K, Oscier DG, et al: Comparison of cytogenetic and restriction fragment length polymorphism analyses for the detection of loss of chromosome material in clonal hemopoietic disorders. *Am J Hematol* 42:171–176, 1993.

Baurmann H, Cherif D, Berger R: Interphase cytogenetics by fluorescent in situ hybridization (FISH) for characterization of monosomy-7-associated myeloid disorders. *Leukemia* 7:384–391, 1993.

Benitez J, Frejo CM, Toledo C, et al: Leukemic transformation in patients with the 5q− alteration: Analysis of the behavior of the 5q− clones in preleukemic to leukemic phases. *Cancer Genet Cytogenet* 26:199–207, 1987.

Berger R, Bernheim A, Daniel MT, et al: Leucemies "induites." Aspects cytogenetique et cytologique. Comparasion avec des leucemies primitives. *Nouvelle Rev Fr Hematol* 23:275–284, 1981.

Bloomfield CD: Chromosome abnormalities in secondary myelodysplastic syndromes. Scand J Haematol 36(Suppl 45):82–90, 1986.

Chen Z, Morgan R, Stone JF, et al: FISH: A useful technique in the verification of clonality of random chromosome abnormalities. *Cancer Genet Cytogenet* 66:73–74, 1993.

Clark SC, Kamen R: The human hematopoietic colony-stimulating factors. *Science* 236:1229–1237, 1987.

Coiffier B, Adeleine P, Viala JJ, et al: Dysmyelopoietic syndromes. A search for prognostic factors in 193 patients. *Cancer* 52:83–90, 1983.

Davis MP, Dewald GW, Pierre RV, et al: Hematologic manifestations associated with deletions of the long arm of chromosome 20. *Cancer Genet Cytogenet* 12:63–71, 1984.

Dewald GW, Davis MP, Pierre RV, et al: Clinical characteristics and prognosis of 50 patients with a myeloproliferative syndrome and deletion of part of the long arm of chromosome 5. *Blood* 66:189–197, 1985.

Diaz MO, Le Beau MM, Harden A, et al: Trisomy 8 in human hematologic neoplasia and the c-*myc* and c-*mos* oncogenes. *Leukemia Research* 9:1437–1442, 1985.

Gilchrist DM, Friedman JM, Rogers PC, et al: Myelodysplasia and leukemia syndrome with monosomy 7: A genetic perspective. *Am J Med Genet* 35:437–441, 1990.

Goyert SM, Ferrero E, Rettig WJ, et al: The CD14 monocyte differentiation antigen maps to a region encoding growth factors and receptors. *Science* 239:497–500, 1988.

Han K, Lee W, Harris CP, et al: Quantifying chromosome changes and lineage involvement in myelodysplastic syndrome (MDS) using fluorescent in situ hybridization (FISH). *Leukemia* 8(1):81–6, 1994.

Heim S, Mitelman F: Chromosome abnormalities in the myelodysplastic syndromes. *Clin Haematol* 15:1003–1021, 1986.

Hoo JJ, Szego K, Jones B: Confirmation of centromeric fusion in 7p/1q translocation associated with myelodysplastic syndrome. *Cancer Genet Cytogenet* 64:186–188, 1992.

Horiike S, Taniwaki M, Misawa S, et al: Chromosome abnormalities and karyotypic evolution in 83 patients with myelodysplastic syndrome and predictive value for prognosis. *Cancer* 62:1129–1138, 1988.

Jacobs RH, Cornbleet MA, Vardiman JW, et al: Prognostic implications of morphology and karyotype in primary myelodysplastic syndromes. *Blood* 67:1765–1772, 1986.

Kadam P, Umerani A, Srivastava A, et al: Combination of classical and interphase cytogenetics to investigate the biology of myeloid disorders: Detection of masked monosomy 7 in AML. *Leuk Res* 17:365–374, 1993.

Kere J, Ruutu T, Lahtinen R, et al: Molecular characterization of chromosome 7 long arm deletions in myeloid disorders. *Blood* 70:1349–1353, 1987.

Kerkhofs H, Hagemeijer A, Leeksma CH, et al: The 5a− chromosome abnormality in hematological disorders: A collaborative study of 34 cases form the Netherlands. *Br J Haematol* 52:365–381, 1982.

Kibbelaar RE, Mulder JW, Dreef EJ, et al: Detection of monosomy 7 and trisomy 8 in myeloid neoplasia: A comparison of banding and fluorescence in situ hybridization. *Blood* 82:904–913, 1993.

Knapp RH, Dewald GW, Pierre RV: Cytogenetic studies in 174 consecutive patients with preleukemic or myelodysplastic syndromes. *Mayo Clin Proc* 60:507–516, 1985.

Kobayashi H, Espinosa R, Fernald A, et al: Analysis of deletions of the long arm of chromosome 11 in hematologic malignancies with fluorescence in situ hybridization. *Genes, Chromosomes Cancer* 8:246–252, 1993.

Le Beau MM: Cytogenetic and molecular analysis of the del(5q) in myeloid disorders: Evidence of the involvement of colony-stimulating factor and FMS genes. In Gale RP, Golde DW (eds): *Recent Advances in Leukemia and Lymphoma*, Vol. 61, New York, Alan R Liss, 1987, pp 71–81.

Le Beau MM, Albain KS, Lason RA, et al: Clinical and cytogenetic correlations in 63 patients with therapy related myelodysplastic syndromes and acute non-lymphocytic leukemia: Further evidence for characteristic abnormalities of chromosome no. 5 and 7. *J Clin Oncol* 4:325–345, 1986.

Le Beau MM, Espinosza R 3d, Neuman WL, et al: Cytogenetic and molecular delineation of the smallest commonly deleted region of chromosome 5 in malignant myeloid diseases. *Proc Natl Acad Sci USA* 90:5484–5488, 1993.

Le Beau MM, Westbrook CA, Diaz MO, et al: *c-src* is consistently conserved in the chromosomal deletion (20q) observed in myeloid disorders. *Proc Natl Acad Sci USA* 82:6692–6696, 1985.

Levine EG, Bloomfield CD: Secondary myelodysplastic syndromes and leukaemias. *Clin Haematol* 15:1037–1080, 1986.

Linman JW, Saarni MI: The preleukemic syndrome. *Semin Hematol* 11:93–100, 1974.

Maschek H, Kaloutsi V, Rodriguez-Kaiser M, et al: Hypoplastic myelodysplastic syndrome: Incidence, morphology, cytogenetics and prognosis. *Ann Hematol* 66:117–122, 1993.

Menke DM, Colon-Otero G, Corkerill KJ, et al: Refractory thrombocytopenia: A myelodysplastic syndrome that may mimic immune thrombocytopenic purpura (see comments). *Am J Clin Pathol* 98:473–475, 1992.

Michiels JJ, Mallios-Zorbala H, Prins MEF, et al: Simple monosomy 7 and myelodysplastic syndrome in thirteen patients without previous cytostatic treatment. *Br J Haematol* 64:425–433, 1986.

Mitelman F, Levan G: Clustering of aberrations to specific chromosomes in human neoplasms. IV. A survey of 1,871 cases. *Hereditas* 95:79–139, 1981.

Morel P, Hebbar M, Lai J-L, et al: Cytogenetic analysis has strong independent prognostic value in de novo myelodysplastic syndromes and can be incorporated in a new scoring system: A report on 408 cases. *Leukemia* 7:1315–1323, 1993.

Morgan R, Hecht F: Deletion of chromosome band 13q14: A primary event in preleukemia and leukemia. *Cancer Genet Cytogenet* 18:243–249, 1985.

Morris SW, Valentine MD, Shapiro DN, et al: Reassignment of the human CSF1 gene to chromosome 1p13–p21. *Blood* 78:2013–2020, 1991.

Mufti GJ: Chromosomal deletions in the myelodysplastic syndrome. *Leuk Res* 16:35–41, 1992.

Mufti GJ, Stevens JR, Oscier DG, et al: Myelodysplastic syndromes: A scoring system with prognostic significance. *Br J Haematol* 59:425–433, 1984.

Nagarajan L, Zavadil J, Claxton D, et al: Consistent loss of the D5S89 locus mapping telomeric to the interleukin gene cluster and centromeric to EGR-1 in patients with 5q− chromosome. *Blood* 83(1):199–208, 1994.

Nair R, Athale UA, Iyer RS, et al: Childhood myelodysplastic syndromes: Clinical features, cytogenetics and prognosis. *Ind J Pediatr* 59:443–448, 1992.

Novak A, Jankovic G, Rolovic Z: Two karyotypically unrelated clones with the t(5;17) and deletion of 5q in myelodysplastic syndrome. *Cancer Genet Cytogenet* 62:100–102, 1992.

Nowell PC, Besa EC, Stelmach T, et al: Chromosome studies in preleukemic states. I. Prognostic significance of single versus multiple abnormalities. *Cancer* 58:2571–2575, 1986.

Pierre RV, Catovsky D, Mufti GJ, et al: Clinical–cytogenetic correlations in myelodysplasia (preleukemia). *Cancer Genet Cytogenet* 40:149–161, 1989.

Ristola M, Kere J, Ruutu T, et al: Reactive oxygen species of neutrophils form patients with monosomy 7 in the bone marrow: Contradictory chemiluminescence activity by whole blood or by purified cells. *Eur J Haematol* 52(1):28–34, 1994.

Roulston D, Espinosa R, Stoffel M, et al: Molecular genetics of myeloid leukemia: Identification of the commonly deleted segment of chromosome 20. *Blood* 82:3424–3429, 1993.

Saltman DL, Dolganov GM, Warrington JA, et al: A physical map of 15 loci on human chromosome 5q23–q33 by two-color fluorescence in situ hybridization. *Genomics* 16:726–732, 1993.

Second International Workshop on Chromosomes in Leukemia (1979): Chromosomes in preleukemia. *Cancer Genet Cytogenet* 2:108–113, 1980.

Sever CE, Pallavicini MG, Meeker TC, et al: Combined fluorescence in situ hybridization and physical mapping studies confirm a relative gene order of IL5, IL4, IRF-1, IL3/GM-CSF, CDC25c on chromosome 5q31. *Blood* submitted.

Shannon KM, Turhan AG, Chang SS, et al: Familial bone marrow monosomy 7. Evidence that the predisposing locus is not on the long arm of chromosome 7. *J Clin Invest* 84:984–989, 1989.

Suciu S, Kuse R, Weh HJ, et al: Results of chromosome studies and their relation to morphology, course, and prognosis in 120 patients with de novo myelodysplastic syndromes. *Cancer Genet Cytogenet* 44:15–26, 1990.

Sukhatme VP, Cao XM, Chang LC, et al: A zinc finger-encoding gene co-regulated with *c-fos* during growth and differentiation, and after cellular depolarization. *Cell* 53:37–43, 1988.

Sullivan SA, Marsden KA, Lowenthal RM, et al: Circulating CD34+ cells: An adverse prognostic factor in the myelodysplastic syndromes. *Am J Hematol* 39:96–101, 1992.

Third MIC Cooperative Study Group: Recommendations for a morphologic, immunologic and cytogenetic (MIC) working classification of the primary and therapy-related myelodysplastic disorders: Report of the workshop held in Scottsdale, AZ, USA. *Cancer Genet Cytogenet* 32:1–10, 1988.

Todd WM, Pierre RV: Preleukaemia: A long-term prospective study of 326 patients. *Scand J Haematol* 36(Suppl 45):114–120, 1986.

Toyama K, Ohyashiki K, Yoshida Y, et al: Clinical implications of chromosomal abnormalities in 401 patients with myelodysplastic syndromes: A multicentric study in Japan. *Leukemia* 7:499–508, 1993.

Van den Berghe H, Cassiman JJ, David G, et al: Distinct haematological disorder with deletion of long arm of no. 5 chromosome. *Nature* 251:437–438, 1974.

Van den Berghe H, Vermaelen K, Mecucci C, et al: The 5q− anomaly. *Cancer Genet Cytogenet* 17:189–255, 1985.

Weiss K, Stass S, Williams D, et al: Childhood monosomy 7 syndrome: Clinical and in vitro studies. *Leukemia* 1:97–104, 1987.

White AD, Culligan DJ, Hoy TG, et al: Extended cytogenetic follow-up of patients with myelodysplastic syndromes. *Br J Haematol* 81:499–502, 1992.

Willman CL, Sever CE, Pallaviani MG, et al: Deletion of IRF-1, mapping to chromosome 5q31, in human leukemia and preleukemia myelodysplasia. *Science* 259:968–971, 1993.

Yunis JJ, Lobell M, Arnesen MA, et al: Refined chromosome study helps define prognostic subgroups in most patients with primary myelodysplastic syndrome and acute myelogenous leukaemia. *Br J Haematol* 68:189–194, 1988.

Yunis JJ, Rydell RE, Oken MM, et al: Refined chromosome analysis as an independent prognostic indicator in de novo myelodysplastic syndromes. *Blood* 67:1721–1730, 1986.

Zanke B, Squire J, Griesser H, et al: A hematopoietic protein tyrosine phosphatase (HePTP) gene that is amplified and overexpressed in myeloid malignancies maps to chromosome 1q32.1. *Leukemia* 8(2):236–244, 1994.

Zhao L, van-Oort J, Cork A, et al: Comparison between interphase and metaphase cytogenetics in detecting chromosome 7 defects in hematological neoplasias. *Am J Hematol* 43:205–211, 1993.

Review Articles

Berger R, Flandrin G: Chromosomal abnormalities in secondary acute myeloid leukaemia and the myelodysplastic syndromes. In Mufti GJ and Golton DAG (eds): *The Myelodysplastic Syndromes*. New York, Churchill Livingstone, 1992, pp 129–139.

Billstrom R, Nilsson PG, Mitelman F: Cytogenetic analysis in 941 consecutive patients with haematologic disorders. *Scand J Haematol* 37:29–40, 1986.

Borgstrom G: Cytogenetics of the myelodysplastic syndromes. *Scand J Haematol* 36(Suppl 45):74–77, 1986.

Fourth International Workshop on Chromosomes in Leukemia, 1982 (1984): Abnormalities of chromosome 7 resulting in monosomy 7 or in deletion of the long arm (7q−): Review of translocations, breakpoints and associated abnormalities. *Cancer Genet Cytogenet* 11:300–303.

Heim S, Mitelman F: Chromosomal abnormalities in primary myelodysplastic syndromes. In Mufti GJ, Galton DAG (eds): *The Myelodysplastic Syndromes*. London, Churchill Livingstone, 1992, pp 115–128.

Human Gene Mapping 9 (1987): Ninth International Workshop on Human Gene Mapping. *Cytogenet Cell Genet* 46:1–762, 1987.

Mecucci C, Van den Berghe H: Cytogenetics. *Hematol Oncol Clin North Am* 6(3):523–541, 1992.

Noel P, Tefferi A, Pierre RV, et al: Karyotypic analysis in primary myelodysplastic syndromes. *Blood Rev* 7:10–18, 1993.

Nowell PC: Cytogenetics of preleukemia. *Cancer Genet Cytogenet* 5:265–278, 1982.

Pedersen B: Survival of patients with t(1;7)(p11;p11). Report of two cases and review of the literature. *Cancer Genet Cytogenet* 60:53–59, 1992.

Pierre RV, Hagland HC, Noel P, et al: Myelodysplastic syndromes (preleukemia). Mayo Clinic Workshop, Lake Louise and Banff Springs, June 1–5, 1992, Alberta, Canada.

Sandberg AA, Wullich B: Myelodysplastic syndromes: Cytogenetic anomalies and their clinical significance. In Schmalzl F, Mufti GJ (eds): *Myelodysplastic Syndromes.* New York, Springer-Verlag, 1992, pp 165–177.

Second International Workshop on Chromosome in Preleukemia: Chromosomes in preleukemia. *Cancer Genet Cytogenet* 2:108–113, 1980.

Thangavelu M, Le Beau MM: Biological significance of chromosomal abnormalities in the myelodysplastic syndromes: In Mufti GJ, Galton DAG (eds): *The Myelodysplastic Syndromes.* New York, Churchill Livingstone, 1992a, pp 141–149.

Thangavelu M, Le Beau MM: Genetic consequences of chromosomal abnormalities in the myelodysplastic syndromes. In Schmalzl F, Mulfti GJ (eds): *Myelodysplastic Syndromes.* New York, Springer Verlag, 1992b, pp 178–186.

CHAPTER **8**

Molecular Genetics and Cytokines

INTRODUCTION: MOLECULAR GENETICS

Leukemogenesis has been thought for some time to be a multistep process. MDSs represent a preleukemic condition which offers an important model for analyzing some of the early steps involved in the progression to leukemia. With the advent of molecular biological technology, tools have become available to characterize the genetic alterations that cause disorders in the control of cell proliferation, differentiation, and intercellular communication leading to malignant transformation. Emerging from the burgeoning molecular data are genomic lesions that play prominent roles in either the activation of oncogenes or the inactivation of tumor-suppressor genes. In the MDSs, mutations and/or deletions of *RAS* family genes, the *FMS* gene, or the *MPL* gene are prototypes of oncogene alteration, whereas the *p53* gene, the deleted in colorectal carcinoma (*DCC*) gene, and the interferon regulatory factor (*IRF*-1) gene are examples of inactivation or deletion of tumor-suppressor genes. In some neoplasias, many different genes have been identified that mutually contribute to the malignant phenotype. Presented in Fig. 8.1 are the mechanisms of oncogenesis that play a predominant role in the pathogenesis of the MDSs and leukemia.

The MDSs have only recently become the subject of scrutiny at the molecular level, and at present our comprehension of the underlying genetic defects is elementary. However, the MDSs offer an exceptional opportunity to dissect the molecular mechanisms underlying hematopoietic failures that frequently lead to the development of leukemia. Table 8.1 presents the genetic abnormalities that are present in the MDSs and acute leukemias.

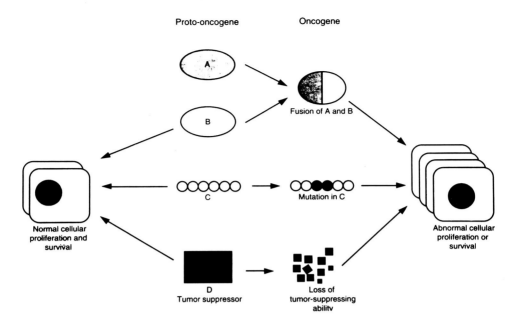

Figure 8.1 Mechanisms of oncogenesis. Normal proto-oncogenes involved in the control of cellular proliferation of survival are converted to cancer-inducing oncogenes as a consequence of either fusion to another gene **(A, B)** or mutation **(C)**. Fusion or mutation results in dysregulated gene expression or an abnormal gene product that causes abnormal proliferation or survival of the host cell. This is usually the first step in the evolution of leukemia. Tumor-suppressor genes **(D)** may be disrupted by mutations, rearrangements, or deletions. The result is loss of their tumor-suppressing gene product, with subsequent abnormal cellular proliferation or survival. This is frequently a secondary event leading to progression to more aggressive forms of leukemia. (From Cline MJ: Mechanisms of disease: The molecular basis of leukemia. *N Engl J Med* 330:328–336, 1994. Reprinted with permission.)

MOLECULAR GENETIC ANALYSIS

Early studies used G6PD isoenzymes as markers to determine the common stem cell origin of granulocytes, erythrocytes, platelets, and lymphocytes in two MDS patients. This strategy was based upon the Lyon hypothesis that only one X chromosome is active in each somatic cell of a female, thus eliminating differences between the sexes in expression of X-linked genes. The inactivation of one X chromosome is random and occurs in early embryogenesis; however, once it occurs, the pattern of X-chromosome inactivation is permanently fixed in all subsequent daughter cells. Therefore, normal female tissue is composed of two cell types: one containing an active, maternally derived, and the other an active, paternally derived X chromosome. However, the studies using G6PD to determine clonality were greatly limited by the rarity of G6PD polymorphisms outside certain ethnic groups.

This restriction was overcome by Vogelstein et al. (1987), who utilized DNA polymorphisms and methylation patterns of X chromosome loci. The maternal and paternal X chromosomes may be distinguished by restriction fragment length polymorphisms (RFLP) using probes for phosphoglycerate kinase (PGK) or hypoxanthine phosphoribosyl transferase (HPRT) genes. Since approximately 50% of females are heterozygous for the PGK and HPRT alleles, these are suitable genes for clonal analysis. The two X chromosomes may be distinguished in more than 90% of females by using a probe, M27 beta, that identifies a variable copy number tandem repeat on the short arm of the X chromosome, designated DXS255. The PCR technology has been applied to study X-chromosome inactivation at the PGK locus and offers the additional advantage of allowing analysis of small cell samples.

Since some healthy females heterozygous for the PGK locus may have a X-inactivation ratio in excess of 80:20 (the usual normal ratio is 50:50), it is most important to include DNA from normal cells before drawing conclusions about the clonality of the tissue under investigation.

Studies performed on 33 patients representing all FAB subtypes heterozygous for PGK and/or HPRT RFLPs by various groups (Bartram, 1992; Gilliland et al., 1991; Janssen et al., 1989; Tefferi et al., 1990) revealed that 30 of them showed a monoclonal pattern of X chromosome inactivation in peripheral blood and bone marrow samples. The X chromosome inactivation analysis was performed in two steps using the PGK probe: (1) the two PGK alleles are first distinguished through RFLP; (2) unmethylated (active) alleles are then cleaved by HpaII. In a monoclonal population, the same PGK allele is active in all cells, and one of the two RFLP fragments is therefore completely lost after HpaII digestion. In contrast, a non-clonal population shows an equal reduction in signal intensity of both RFLP fragments. Recently, Van Kamp et al. (1991) evaluated 11 female heterozygous MDS patients by RFLPs of the X-linked genes *PGK*-1 and *HPRT* with the M27 beta probe. All (three RA, two RARS, two CMML, four RAEB-IT) exhibited clonal hematopoiesis, as determined by Southern blot analysis of DNA prepared from peripheral blood and/or bone marrow cells. In addition, subpopulations of cells were separated by means of a fluorescence-activated cell sorter into polymorpho-nuclear (PMN) cells, monocytes, T and B lymphocytes, and natural killer (NK) cells. They determined by Southern and PCR analysis that PMN cells and mono-cytes were clonally derived, whereas circulating T and B lymphocytes and NK cells exhibited random X-chromosome inactivation compatible with a polyclonal pattern. Therefore, it could be concluded from this study that MDS represents a clonal disorder restricted to cells of myeloid origin.

Sparse data on X-chromosome inactivation in childhood MDS have appeared in the literature. Although the disease closely resembles adult MDS, it shows a similar spectrum of chromosomal abnormalities and can be readily classified according to FAB criteria.

Many diagnostic problems arise in cases of hypoplastic RA and aplastic anemia. X-chromosome inactivation analysis indicates that MDS in children is a clonal disease. However, Tsuge et al. (1993) presented similar data on 4 of 20 female patients with aplastic anemia who responded to antilymphocyte globulin and on follow-up showed no evidence of a clonal disorder such as MDS. These findings limit the diagnostic distinction between hypoplastic MDS and aplastic anemia; nevertheless, they allow new insights into the pathogenesis of aplastic anemia as a possible preleukemic disorder.

In addition to aplastic anemia, difficulties arise in distinguishing between diffi-cult cases of MPD and MDS which have overlapping features. Kreipe (1993),

Table 8.1 Genetic Abnormalities in MDS and Leukemia

Type of Gene	Function	Molecular Alteration	Common Chromosomal Abnormality	Approximate Percentage of MDS and Leukemia with Abnormality
RAS	Signal transduction	N-RAS mutations	None	MDS, 9–40% AML, 15–50% ALL, 14% Blast crisis CML, <5%
Tyrosine kinases	Membrane signal transduction	FMS mutation and deletion Fusion of c-abl to bcr	del 5q t(9;22) (q34;q11)	MDS, 16% AML, 20% ALL, 5–20% CML, >95%
Transcriptional control element	Gene transcription	Fusion of myc to immunoglobulin genes	t(8;14) (q24;q32)	Burkitt's lymphoma, 100% Pre-B-cell ALL, T-ALL, <10%
		Fusion of E2A to PBX or HLF	t(1;19) (q23;p13) t(17;19) (q22;p13)	Pre-B-cell ALL, <10%
		Fusion of SCL (tal-1) to TCR or SIL genes	t(1;14) (p32;q11)	T-ALL, 15–25%
		Fusion of tal-2 to TCR genes Fusion of lyl-1 to TCR genes Fusion of Ttg-1, ttg-2 to TCR genes	t(7;9) (q35;p13) t(17;19) (q35;p13) t(11;14) (p15;q11) t(11;14) (p13;q11)	T-ALL, <10% T-ALL, <5% T-ALL, <10%
Receptor	Differentiation	Fusion of α-retinoic acid-receptor gene to PML	t(15;17) (q21;q21)	Acute promyelocytic leukemia, 100%
	Cytokine receptor signal transduction	MPL amplification	1p34	MDS 31% AML 51%
bcl	Apoptosis, other functions?	Fusion of bcl-2 to immunoglobulin genes	t(14;18) (q32;q21)	Follicular lymphoma, >75% Diffuse lymphoma, 20% CLL, 5%
	Cell-cycle control	Fusion of bcl-1 to immunoglobulin genes	t(11;14) (q13;q32)	Centrocytic lymphoma, >30% CLL, 2–5%
	Inhibition of gene transcription	Fusion of bcl-3 to immunoglobulin genes	t(14;19) (q32;q13)	CLL, <10%

Category	Function	Molecular event	Cytogenetics	Disease association
Homeodomain	Differentiation and gene transcription	Fusion of HOX-11 to TCR genes	t(10;14) (q24;q11)	T-ALL, 7%
Anti-oncogenes	Tumor suppression, transcription, cell-cycle control, apoptosis	HRX translocation	t(11q23)	Multilineage leukemia? MDS, 5%?
		Mutation, loss, or rearrangement of p53	Mutation / del 17	Blast crisis of CML, >20%; AML, 3–7%; Pre-B-cell ALL, 2%; T-ALL, <2%; Burkitt's lymphoma, 30%; CLL, 15%; AML, 3–7%
		Disruption of RBI	13q	Pre-B-cell ALL, 2%; T-ALL, 2%; Burkitt's lymphoma, 30%; CLL, 15%; Ph^1-positive ALL, >30%; AML, <3%; AMML, 25%; Pre-B-cell ALL, T-ALL, 20%
		Loss of WT1	11p	AML, 20%?
		Deletion of IRF-1	5q31.1	MDS-increased, acute leukemia—increased
		Loss of DCC	del 18q	MDS, 8%; MDS → AML, 71%; AML, 31%; ALL, 33%
Other	Function unknown	Fusion DEK/CAN, SET/CAN	t(6;9) (p23;q34)	AML, MDS, <2%
		Fusion of MLL	t(11q33)	AML? ALL?
		Rearrangement of TAN-1	t(7;9) (q34; q34.3)	T-ALL?
		Fusion of AML1	t(8;21)	AML?
	Regulation of growth	Fusion of IL-3	t(5;14) (q31;q32)	Pre-B-cell ALL?

Abbreviations: ALL = acute lymphoblastic leukemia; AML = acute myeloid leukemia; T-ALL = T-cell lymphoblastic leukemia; TCR = T-cell receptor; AMML = acute myelomonocytic leukemia (FAB M4 or M5 AML); MDS's = myelodysplastic syndromes; DCC = deleted in colorectal carcinoma; IRF = interferon regulatory factor.

Source: Cline MJ: Mechanisms of disease: The molecular basis of leukemia. *N Engl J Med* 330:329, 1994; Vigon I, Dreyfus F, Melle J, et al: Expression of the *c-mpl* proto-oncogene in human hematologic malignancies. *Blood* 82:877–882, 1993; Miyake K, Mokuchi K, Dan K, et al: Alterations in the deleted colorectal carcinoma gene in human primary leukemia. *Blood* 82:927–930, 1993; Willman CL, Sever CE, Pallovicini MG, et al: Deletion of *IRF*-1, mapping to chromosome 5q 31.1, in human leukemia and preleukemic myelodysplasia. *Science* 259:968–971, 1993.

using X-chromosome-linked DNA polymorphism in conjunction with methylation patterns, was unable to distinguish MPD cases from MDS cases since both exhibited clonal hematopoiesis. Nevertheless, despite morphological overlap between different types of MPD and MDS, the presence of *bcr* gene rearrangement proved to be specific for CML, and could be applied to differentiate CML from MPD cases of difficult and uncertain morphological diagnosis.

Recently, FISH has been employed to detect clonality of the MDSs. Anastasi et al. (1993), using FISH with a probe for the centromere of chromosome 8, identified trisomy 8 in individual peripheral blood cells in Wright-stained smears. Also, Chen et al. (1992), using FISH and centromere probes for chromosomes 1, 6, 7, 8, 9, 12, 18, 13/21, and X, determined clonality in the MDSs and leukemias. Thus, additional techniques have become available to establish clonality in MDSs and the leukemias.

Finally, an intriguing study by Jowitt et al. (1993) utilized X-chromosome-linked RFLP to analyze clonality in a female with AML. The results demonstrated that the initial MDS clone was genotypically distinct from the MDS clone that emerged following treatment of her AML. The authors believe that such a switch in clonality after evolution through an episode of AML allows new insights into the biology and origin of AML. These observations support a multistep hypothesis for the development of MDS in its progression to leukemia.

RAS MUTATIONS

Somatic mutations of *RAS* proto-oncogenes is one of the most common genetic alterations found in primary and experimentally induced tumors. The suggestion that *RAS* mutations may constitute an important event in the development of human myeloid leukemia originated with the discovery of transforming *RAS* genes in de novo AML and in myeloid cell lines. Such findings have also now been extended to the MDSs.

RAS genes form part of a multigene family, the most widely studied of which include H-, K-, and N-*RAS* (Table 8.2). *RAS* genes encode highly related 21-kd proteins that play a pivotal role in the transduction of growth and differentiation stimuli. Despite being the focus of enormous scientific interest, the function of RAS proteins remains enigmatic. Nevertheless, it is known that $p21^{RAS}$ and the α-unit of G proteins demonstrate structural and functional homology. The G proteins, a family of guanine-nucleotide binding proteins, are necessary components in signal transduction pathways derived from activated cell surface receptors. Therefore, such findings suggest that RAS proteins play a role in growth factor–regulated transmembrane signaling. In support of such a function is the fact that RAS proteins are anchored to the inner surface of the cell membrane and, in their basal state, are complexed with guanosine diphosphate (GDP). Since RAS proteins possess GDP- and guanosine triphosphate (GTP)-binding capabilities as well as intrinsic GTPase properties, regulation of their biological activity is controlled by hydrolysis of $p21^{RAS}$. This reaction promotes an interaction of $p21^{RAS}$ with putative effector molecules, resulting in the generation of a mitotic signal. Recently, two proteins that interact with $p21^{RAS}$ have been identified: GAP (GTPase-activating

Table 8.4   *FMS* Mutations in MDS Patients

	No. of Patients	*FMS Mutations*		
		301	*969*	*Total*
RA	27	—	4	4 (14%)
RARS	20	1	—	1 (5%)
RAEB/RAEB-IT	21	0	2	2 (9%)
CMML	40	1	10	11 (27%)
Totals	108	2	16	18 (16%)

Source: Bartram CR: Molecular genetic aspects of myelodysplastic syndromes. *Hematol Oncol Clin North Am* 6:563, 1992.

of patients. *FMS* mutations in MDS patients compiled by Bartram are shown in Table 8.4.

Although the FMS mutations and deletions may be of minor importance in leukemogenesis, a remarkable number of growth factors and growth factor receptor genes reside on the long arm of chromosome 5 in the region 5q11–q33 (see Chapter 7). These include IL-3, IL-4, IL-5, IRF-1 (interferon regulatory factor-1), M-CSF, GM-CSF, and CDC25C. Recently, Willman et al. have shown that the *IRF-1* gene at 5q31.1 was consistently deleted in 13 cases of leukemia and myelodysplasia (Fig. 8.3). However, cases have been reported by other investigators that did not show the *IRF-1* gene deletion.

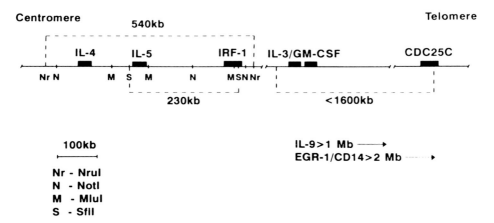

Figure 8.3   Physical map of the 5q31 chromosome region generated by a combination of pulse-field gel electrophoresis and multicolor FISH techniques. Boxes represent coding exons of IL-4, IL-5, IRF-1, IL-3, GM-CSF, and CDC25C. Although this map is most important and of great interest, it is now agreed that the *IRF-1* gene is not the major gene in MDS and myeloid leukemia pathogenesis. Currently, the critical region is believed to be more distal on q31. (Courtesy of Cheryl L. Willman, Linda M. Boxer, and Michael L. Cleary.)

MPL AMPLIFICATION

Similarly to two other hematopoietic growth factor receptors, the *FMS* and *KIT* genes, the *MPL* gene was discovered through the study of oncogenic retroviruses. However, unlike *FMS* and *KIT* genes that encode a subgroup of tyrosine kinase receptors, the *MPL* proto-oncogene encodes a new member of a cytokine receptor superfamily. Although levels of *MPL* transcripts in lymphoid malignancies and chronic myeloproliferative disorders were not significantly different from those in normal marrow cells, Vigon et al. have shown that *MPL* expression was increased in 26 of 51 patients with acute myeloblastic leukemia and in 5 of 16 patients with MDSs. There was no correlation between amplification of the *MPL* gene and the FAB classification of AML. Nevertheless, patients with high *MPL* expression appeared to belong to a subgroup of AML patients with a low rate of complete remission and a poor prognosis, including those with secondary leukemia and AML with unfavorable cytogenetic abnormalities.

TUMOR-SUPPRESSOR GENES

Some neoplasias have biallelic alterations that result in loss of gene function. Such genes are called *tumor-suppressor genes* or *recessive oncogenes*. Normally, their products down regulate growth and differentiation and indirectly protect against malignant transformation. With the use of cytogenetic analysis, DNA polymorphisms, Southern blot analysis, pulsed-field gel electrophoresis, computer-assisted fluorescence microscopic analysis, and chromosomal FISH, investigators have been able to identify respective loci that have been inactivated or deleted. Since MDSs are frequently associated with chromosomal deletions, it would seem logical to think that some of the deleted regions probably contain tumor-suppressor genes. Currently, a number of tumor-suppressor genes have been implicated in the MDSs. These include p53, the *DCC* gene, and the *IRF*-1 gene.

p53 Mutations

Point mutations in the p53 tumor-suppressor gene located on chromosome 17 are the most frequently identified genetic alterations in human malignancies. Inactivation of p53 is also observed in AML patients.

Recently, Sugimoto et al. (1993) evaluated 44 patients with MDS and with overt leukemia that evolved from MDS for p53 alterations, using reverse transcriptase-PCR, single-stranded conformation analysis, and nucleotide sequencing. Three patients with MDS (two RAEB and one RAEB-IT) had point mutations in the conserved regions of the p53 coding sequence. Expression of the wild-type p53 mRNA was not detected in any of these three patients. Interestingly, the three MDS patients with the p53 gene mutations showed no N-*RAS* gene mutations, suggesting heterogeneity in the oncogenic mechanism of MDS. Ludwig et al. (1992) had similar findings in evaluating 61 patients with MDS using single-stranded conformation polymorphism analysis of PCR products as well as direct sequencing. They found p53 mutations in only 1 of 14 RAEB patients and 2 of 5

RAEB-IT patients. The three mutations represented G:C to A:T transitions at codon 141 (exon 5) and codons 245 and 248 (exon 7), respectively. Therefore, from these studies and others, one can conclude that p53 mutations may contribute, albeit rarely, to the development of preleukemic disorders of the myeloid cell lineage.

DCC Gene

The *DCC* gene on chromosome 18q encodes a protein with significant sequence similarity to the neural cell adhesion molecule and other related cell surface glycoproteins. Alteration of this gene may interfere with normal cell growth and differentiation by disrupting cell–cell or cell–substrate interactions. Recently, Miyake et al. (1993b) evaluated the expression of the *DCC* gene in MDSs and overt leukemia by means of reverse transcriptase-PCR analysis. They used the reverse transcriptase-PCR in 24 MDS cases and in 7 overt leukemia cases that progressed from MDS. Surprisingly, the expression of the *DCC* gene was absent or extremely reduced in 2 of the 24 MDS patients, and those 2 patients developed overt leukemia within 6 months. Moreover, in five of the seven cases of overt leukemia that developed from MDS, expression of the *DCC* gene was absent or extremely reduced. The authors suggest that inactivation of the *DCC* gene may be the late event that triggers the progression of MDS to leukemia. Additional studies by other investigators are needed to support this most interesting finding.

Interferon Regulatory Factor-1

Among the most frequent cytogenetic abnormalities in human MDSs and leukemia is an interstitial deletion within the long arm of chromosome 5 [del(5q) or "5q−"]. Del(5q) was initially described as the hallmark of a unique MDS with RA designated the *5q− syndrome*. This distinctive karyotypic finding occurs in 30% of patients with MDS, as well as in 50% of patients with AML arising secondary to MDS or prior chemotherapy, in 15% of de novo AMLs, and in 2% of de novo acute lymphocytic leukemias. Although the proximal and distal breakpoints of del(5q) vary from patient to patient, the smallest commonly deleted segment is band 5q31. Further, rare de novo AMLs with translocations of 5q31 have been described. With this background, a tumor-suppressor gene has been postulated to lie in the 5q31 region.

Recently, Willman et al. (1993) have mapped the gene encoding interferon regulatory factor-1 (IRF-1) to chromosome 5q31.1 (Fig. 8.2). This protein, which functions as a transcriptional activator of interferon (IFN) α, β, and other IFN-inducible genes, has recently been found to possess growth inhibitory and antioncogenic activities. The *IRF*-1 gene lies between IL-5 and CDC25C and is centromeric to IL-3 and GM-CSF (see Chapter 7). Among all of the genes in this region, only *IRF*-1 was consistently deleted at one or both alleles in 13 cases of leukemia or MDS with abnormalities of 5q31. However, Boultwood et al. (1993) recently showed that 2 of 14 MDS and AML patients with deletions involving 5q31 had retained both copies of the *IRF*-1 gene. Also, Kroef et al. (1994) reported two additional cases that have both *IRF*-1 alleles despite the presence of 5q31 deletions. Although *IRF*-1 is not consistently lost in every patient with the 5q31 deletion, the above findings do not exclude *IRF*-1 as the responsible tumor suppressor, since inactivation of both alleles could still have occurred by two independent point mutations. Detailed characterization of the *IRF*-1 coding regions by single-stranded conformation polymorphism–based screening methods and sequence analysis should provide the insight needed to determine the potential role of the *IRF*-1 gene in the MDSs and leukemias.

Apparently, unusual instability exists in the 5q region. This instability, rather than mutations, may be responsible for the observed deletions or rearrangements within this region.

FUTURE DIRECTIONS

It is becoming increasingly clear that our understanding of the disruption of cell proliferation, differentiation, and intercellular communication in leukemogenesis will come through molecular biology. Current evidence indicates that activation of oncogenes and inactivation of tumor-suppressor genes play an important role in both myelodysplasia and leukemia. Mutations of *RAS* and *FMS* genes activate oncogenes; alteration of the *p-53* gene and deletions of the *DCC* and *IRF*-1 genes release tumor suppression and support malignant growth. Current evidence seems to indicate that the critical region involved in the MDSs and leukemias resides in the critical region distal to the *IRF*-1 gene. Therefore, this critical region will need to be studied in greater detail to determine its crucial contribution to the production of MDSs and leukemia. New oncogenes, tumor-suppressor genes, apoptotic genes, MHC expression genes, and signal transduction genes need to be discovered, studied, and integrated into our current knowledge of the molecular genetics of the MDSs and leukemias.

INTRODUCTION: CYTOKINES

The mechanisms that control growth, differentiation, and division of hematopoietic cells remain poorly understood. In the 1960s, culture techniques utilizing semisolid microenvironments were developed that successfully supported the clonal growth of normal hematopoietic progenitor cells. Such systems added greatly to previous, more cumbersome, in vivo assays of hematopoiesis, such as injecting hematopoietic cells into lethally irradiated mice and surveying their spleens for the appearance of hematopoietic colonies.

With the arrival of these in vitro systems, it was shown that specific glycoproteins are required for the survival, proliferation, and induction of lineage-specific differentiation in both normal and leukemic cells. Initially, growth factors defined on the myeloid differentiation pathways were termed *colony-stimulating factors (CSFs)*, and those defined generally on lymphoid pathways were designated *interleukins (ILs)*. However, as information accumulated, it became increasingly obvious that CSFs, ILs, and oncogenes are inextricably intertwined in cell growth, differentiation, and division. Indeed, even other cytokines not originally identified by their effects on hematopoietic cells, such as tumor necrosis factor and transforming growth factor-beta, may also have important regulatory effects on hematopoiesis.

Cytokines: Location and Function

A number of hematopoietic factors have been identified, purified, and cloned by molecular recombinant techniques, thus enabling the production of these hematopoietic hormones in quantities sufficient for preclinical studies and for clinical application. They include erythropoietin (Ep), a physiological regulator of erythropoiesis; granulocyte-macrophage colony-stimulating factor (GM-CSF); granulocyte colony-stimulating factor (G-CSF); IL-3 granulocyte-erythrocyte-macrophage-megakaryocyte, (GEMM); macrophage colony-stimulating factor (M-CSF); IL-4, IL-5, IL-6, and IL-11; and IFN-α, IFN-β and IFN-γ. The major growth factors are presented in Table 8.5.

A high incidence of genes for growth factors and growth factor receptors occurs on the long arm of chromosome 5 (Figs. 7.2, 8.3). Deletions in the long arm of chromosome 5 are also frequently associated with the development of myeloid abnormalities and acute leukemias. One such disorder, the 5q− syndrome, is characterized by macrocytic anemia and deletion of the region 5q31.

With the exception of Ep, the physiological roles of these factors have not yet been clearly established. However, in general (to name only a few important functions), GM-CSF stimulates granulocyte-macrophage, granulocyte, and macrophage colony factor formation in vitro and proliferation of normal human promyelocytes and myelocytes. G-CSF stimulates formation of granulocyte colonies in vitro and some granulocyte-macrophage progenitors, but the latter are not sustained beyond a few days. IL-3 (GEMM), also called *multi-CSF*, stimulates formation of the granulocyte, macrophage, eosinophil, mast cell, NK-like cell, and erythroid and multipotent colonies from murine fetal liver and bone marrow. M-CSF, CSF-1, stimulates predominantly macrophage colonies in vitro with some granulocyte component early in culture. IL-4, or B-cell stimulating factor, acts as a costimulant with anti-IgM antibodies for entry of resting B cells into DNA synthesis and increased expression of class II MHC molecules on resting B cells. IL-5 promotes IgM secretion and proliferation by *BCL*-1 B-cell lines, induces hapten-specific IgG secretion in vitro by in vivo antigen-primed B cells, and promotes differentiation of normal B cells. It also stimulates eosinophil colony formation and differentiation in liquid culture. IL-6 has the ability to enhance Ig secretion by B lymphocytes and to induce B cells. It also supports growth of Epstein-Barr virus–infected B cells.

IL-7, a stromal cell–derived cytokine, stimulates DNA synthesis in ALL cells of B- and T-cell precursor origin. Apparently, IL-7 is involved in the complex regulation of ALL cell production. How it relates to the ALL blast crisis of CML remains to be investigated.

IL-8, a keratinocyte-derived molecule, also known as *neutrophil attractant-activation protein* (NAP-1), attracts and activates human neutrophils but is not a chemoattractant for human monocytes. The role of IL-8, especially in CML, remains to be elucidated.

IL-9 has a genomic sequence homology with a human IL-9 cDNA isolated from HTLV-I-transformed T cells by expression cloning. The *IL-9* gene has been mapped to the long arm of chromosome 5 at band 5q31–32, a region found to be deleted in a number of patients with acquired 5q− abnormalities and hematological disorders. The 5′ regulatory region of the human *IL-9* gene also contains sequences

Table 8.5 Growth Factors

Cytokines	Cell Sources	Functions

IL-1	Monocytes-macrophages
	B cells
	Epithelial cells
	Fibroblasts, astrocytes
	Dendritic cells
	Keratinocytes
		Endogenous pyrogen
		Growth factor for
		  lymphocytes, fibroblasts,
		  synovial cells, endothelial
		  cells, hematopoietic cells
		Induction of acute-phase
		  proteins

IL-2	Activated T cells	Growth and differentiation factor
		  for lymphocytes and
		  endothelial cells

IL-3, G-CSF,
  GM-CSF,
  M-CSF
	Monocytes
	T cells
		Growth factors for hematopoietic
		  cells

IL-4	Activated T-cells	Growth and differentiation factor for lymphocytes
IL-5	T cells	Eosinophil growth factor, B-cell differentiation factor

IL-6	Monocytes-macrophages
	B cells
	Epithelial cells
	Fibroblasts, astrocytes
	Dendritic cells
	Keratinocytes
		Endogenous pyrogen
		Growth factor for lymphocytes,
		  fibroblasts, synovial cells,
		  endothelial cells,
		  hematopoietic cells
		Induction of acute phase
		  proteins
		Plasma cell growth factor

IL-7	Bone marrow stroma cells Spleen cells	Growth factor of pre-B and pre-T lymphocytes
IL-8	Monocytes T lymphocytes	Neutrophil chemotactic factor
IL-9	T lymphocytes	T-cell growth factor
IL-10	T lymphocytes	T-helper cell inhibitory factor Stem cell growth factor
IL-11	Stromal cells	Multifunctional regulator of hematopoiesis

IL-12	Human B lymphoblastoid
	  cell line (NC-37)
		Functional activation of NK cells
		Induction of LAK cells
		  synergistically with IL-2
		Augmentation of allogeneic CTL
		  response
		Enhancement of IL-2-induced
		  proliferation of resting
		  peripheral blood cells

IL-13	Th 2 cells	Induces proliferation, Ig isotype
		  switching, and Ig synthesis
		Down modulates macrophage
		  activity
		Induces IgE synthesis

IL-14	T cells	Induces B-cell proliferation

Table 8.5 (continued)

Cytokines	Cell Sources	Functions
	Some malignant B cells	Inhibits immunoglobulin secretion Selectively expands certain B-cell populations
IL-15	Epithelial and fibroblast cell lines Adherent peripheral blood mononuclear cells	Stimulates proliferation of IL-2-dependent cell line and activated peripheral blood T cells Induces generation of cytolytic effector cells in vitro
IFN-α	Buffy coat leukocytes Namaliva cells KG-1 cells Akube cells B lymphocytes CML cells Fibroblasts induced by viruses	Inhibition of growth of tumor cells Stimulation of NK cell activity Stimulation of cytotoxic T cells and macrophages

IFN-β	Fibroblasts
	Some epithelial cells, such as amniotic cells
	Osteosarcoma MG63
	Embryonic tissue
	Breast carcinosarcoma
		Increases cell surface
		  Cell surface HLA class I and II antigen
		  Serum B$_2$-microglobulin
		  Serum neopterin
		  NK activity
		  Lymphocyte CD38 reactivity
		  2,5 A synthetase activity in peripheral blood lymphocytes
		  Antibody-dependent cellular cytotoxicity

IFN-δ	T and NK cells	Antiviral activity antiproliferative activity on tumor cells Induction of MHC class I and II antigens Activates macrophages to become tumoricidal and kill intracellular parasites Enhances NK cell activity Induces immunoglobulin secretion by B cells and enhances B-cell motivation and proliferation Inhibits osteoclast activation
Interferon (IFN)	T and NK cells	Differentiation factor for B cells Activator of NK cells and macrophages

Table 8.5 (continued)

Cytokines	Cell Sources	Functions
Tumor necrosis factor (TNF) α/β	Monocytes T cells	Antivirus Cytotoxic factor Cachectin Septic shock Growth factor for hematopoietic and fibroblastic cells

Source: Friedman WH: Pathophysiology of cytokines. *Leuk Res* 14(8):675–677, 1990; Pumonen PJ, de-Vries JE: IL-13 induces proliferation, Ig isotype switching, and Ig synthesis by immature human fetal B cells. *J Immunol* 152:1094–1102, 1994; Ambrus JL Jr., Pippin J, Joseph A, et al: Identification of a cDNA for a human high-molecular weight B-cell growth factor. *Proc Natl Acad Sci USA* 90:6330–6334, 1993; Grabstein KH, Eisenman J, Shanebeck K, et al: Cloning of a T cell growth factor that interacts with the B chain of the interleukin-2 receptor. *Science* 264:965–968, 1994.

identified in the 5' flanking regions of other cytokine genes mapped to the long arm of chromosome 5, including IL-3, IL-4, IL-5, and GM-CSF and other T-cell growth factor genes, including IL-2 and IL-6. The *IL-9* gene is constitutively expressed in the HTLV-I-transformed human T cells, and the expression of *IL-9* in these cells can be further induced by 12-9-tetradecanoyl-phorbol-13-acetate. Undoubtedly, understanding of *IL-9* gene expression will allow us to study the regulatory mechanisms in normal and leukemic human T cells.

IL-10 exhibits strong DNA and amino acid sequence homology to an open reading frame in the Epstein-Barr virus, BCRFI. Both human IL-10 and the BCRFI product inhibit cytokine synthesis by activated human peripheral blood mononuclear cells. Also, both human and mouse IL-10 sustain the viability of a mouse mast cell line in culture. Therefore, this cytokine has implications for the modulation of mastocytosis and mast cell leukemia.

IL-11, a stromal cell–derived cytokine, is capable of stimulating plasmacytoma proliferation and T-cell-dependent development of Ig-reproducing B cells; it also synergizes with IL-3 in supporting murine megakaryocyte colony formation. These properties implicate IL-11 as an additional multifunctional regulator in the hematopoietic microenvironment.

IL-12 is a cytokine which, like IFN-γ and IFN-α, may be involved in conferring protective immunity against infectious agents such as viruses. Previously known as *natural killer cell stimulatory factor* or *cytotoxic lymphocyte maturation factor*, IL-12 is a 75-kD heterodimeric glycoprotein displaying several in vitro activities, including (1) enhancement in synergy with IL-2; (2) increase in the cytotoxic activity of NK cells; (3) promotion of the proliferation of activated T and NK cells; and (4) induction of IFN-γ production by resting or activated peripheral blood T and NK cells.

IL-13 is a neoteric T-cell-derived cytokine that induces proliferation, Ig isotype switching, and Ig synthesis by human immature B cells derived from fetal bone marrow. It is produced in Th2 cells and is also capable of down-modulating macrophage activity in a manner similar to that previously described for IL-4. Furthermore, it can inhibit inflammatory cytokine production by lipopolysaccharide-activated monocytes. The protein encoded by IL-13 cDNA is the human homologue of a mouse Th2 product called p600. Apparently, IL-13 acts at different stages of the B-cell maturation pathway in that it enhances the expression of CD23/Fc epsilon RII and class II MHC antigens on resting B cells; it stimulates B-cell proliferation in combination with anti-Ig and anti-CD40 antibodies; and it induces IgE synthesis. Thus, the spectrum of the biological activities of IL-13 on B cells largely overlaps that previously ascribed to IL-4.

IL-14 is a novel high molecular weight B-cell growth factor. Purified IL-14 has been shown to induce B-cell proliferation, inhibit immunoglobulin secretion, and selectively expand certain B-cell subpopulations. Studies using antibodies to IL-14 and its receptor have suggested that IL-14, while produced by T cells and some malignant B cells, acts predominately on normal and malignant B cells. IL-14 cDNA has been identified by Ambrus et al. (1993) by expression cloning using a moAb and polyclonal antisera to IL-14. The protein produced in the cDNA induced B-cell proliferation, inhibited immunoglobulin secretion, and was recognized in immunoblots by anti-IL-14 antibodies. The amino acid sequence of the IL-14 deduced from the cDNA predicts a 53-kD secreted protein with three potential N-linked glycosylation sites. Currently, studies are in progress to further characterize the physiological roles of this new cytokine.

IL-15 was recently discovered in the course of testing supernatants from a simian kidney epithelial cell line for cytokine activity. It was discovered that these cells produced a soluble factor capable of supporting proliferation of an IL-2-dependent cell line, CTLL. Although IL-2 and IL-15 show no sequence similarity, they show many structural similarities which are characteristic of a helical cytokine family.

IL-15 demonstrates biological activity resembling that of IL-2, which also uses components of the IL-2 receptor. In addition to stimulating proliferation of the CTLL cell line and activated peripheral blood T cells, IL-15, like IL-2, induces the generation of cytolytic effector cells in vitro.

Although some activities are shared by IL-2 and IL-15, there are also differences between the biological effects of these two cytokines.

FUTURE DIRECTIONS

Advances in our understanding of the cytokine network will most likely come from cytokine gene knockout mice and mice transgenic for cytokine gene reporter constructs, particularly when acute or chronic infections, autoimmune processes, or neoplasia are induced in either type of animal. In situ studies of mRNA and protein of a range of cytokines and their receptors in human development, tissue repair, infection, inflammation, and cancer should also contribute to our understanding. Also, in vitro actions of cytokines can provide useful indications of in vivo action. Some, if not all, of the in vivo behavior of cytokines, such as CSF, IL-3, IL-6, and IL-2 could have been predicted from in vitro studies. Such a systemic analysis of all new and existing cytokines will continue to provide useful information and generate new ideas concerning the cytokines in the MDSs and the leukemias. This information will undoubtedly provide a new and better treatment armamentarium for these disorders.

BIBLIOGRAPHY

Articles

Anastasi J, Feng J, Le Beau MM et al: Cytogenetic clonality in myelodysplastic syndromes studied with fluorescence in situ hybridization: Lineage, response to growth factor therapy, and clone expansion. *Blood* 81:1580–1585, 1993.

Ardern JC, Saunders MJ, Hyde K, et al: Polymerase chain reaction analysis of allele frequency and loss at the Harvey ras locus in myeloid malignancies. *Leukemia* 7:258–262, 1993.

Ballester R, Michaeli T, Ferguson K, et al: Genetic analysis of mammalian GAP expressed in yeast. *Cell* 59:681–686, 1989.

Bishop JM: Molecular themes in oncogenesis. *Cell* 64:235–248, 1991.

Boultwood J, Fidler C, Lewis S, et al: Allelic loss of IRF1 in myelodysplasia and acute myeloid leukemia: Retention of IRF1 on the 5q-chromosome in some patients with the 5q-syndrome. *Blood* 82:2611–2616, 1993.

Brodeur GM: The *NF1* gene in myelopoiesis and childhood myelodysplastic syndromes. *N Engl J Med* 330:637–638, 1994.

Brown RM, Fraser NJ, Brown GK: Differential methylation of the hypervariable locus DXS 255 on active and inactive X-chromosomes correlates with the expression of a human X-linked gene. *Genomics* 7:215–221, 1990.

Carter G, Hughes DC, Clark RE, et al: *RAS* mutations in patients following cytotoxic therapy for lymphoma. *Oncogene* 5:411–416, 1990.

Chen Z, Morgan R, Berger CS, et al: Application of fluorescence in situ hybridization in hematological disorders. *Cancer Genet Cytogenet* 63:62–69, 1992.

Fearon ER, Vogelstein B: A genetic model for colorectal tumorigenesis. *Cell* 61:759–767, 1990.

Feng BZ, Lei JL, Yang XY: Gene diagnosis and successful reversion in a patient with preleukemia. *Chung-Hua-Nei-Ko-Tsa-Chil* 31:539–542, 1992.

Fraser NJ, Boyd Y, Brownlee GG, et al: Multi-allelic RFLP for M27Beta, an anonymous single copy genomic clone at Xp/11.3- Xcen [HGM9 provisional no. DX5255]. *Nucl Acids Res* 15:9616, 1987.

Gambke C, Hall A, Moroni C: Activation of an *N*-ras gene in acute myeloblastic leukemia through somatic mutation in the first exon. *Proc Natl Acad Sci USA* 82:879–882, 1985.

Gilliland DG, Blanchard KL, Levy J, et al: Clonality in myeloproliferative disorders: Analysis by means of the polymerase chain reaction. *Proc Natl Acad Sci USA* 88:6848–6852, 1991.

Golub TR, Barker GF, Lovett M, et al: Fusion of PDGF receptor β to a novel *ets*-like gene, *tel*, in chronic myelomonocytic leukemia with t(5;12) chromosomal translocation. Cell 77:307–318, 1994.

Hirai H, Okada M, Mizoguchi H, et al: Relationship between an activated N-*ras* oncogene and chromosomal abnormality during leukemic progression from myelodysplastic syndrome. *Blood* 71:256–258, 1988.

Hodges E, Howell WM, Boyd Y, et al: Variable x-chromosome DNA methylation patterns detected with probe M27*B* in a series of lymphoid and myeloid malignancies. *Br J Haematol* 77:315–322, 1991.

Hunter T: Cooperation between oncogenes. *Cell* 64:249–270, 1991.

Janssen JW, Buschle M, Layton M, et al: Clonal analysis of myelodysplastic syndromes: Evidence of multipotent stem cell origin. *Blood* 73:248–254, 1989.

Janssen JW, Lyons J, Steenvoorden ACM, et al: Concurrent mutations in two different *ras* genes in acute myelocytic leukemias. *Nucl Acid Res* 15:5669–5680, 1987.

Jowitt SN, Yin JA, Saunders MJ: Relapsed myelodysplastic clone differs from acute onset clone as shown by X-linked DNA polymorphism patterns with acute myeloid leukemia. *Blood* 82:613–618, 1993.

Kalmantis T, Kalmanti M, Vassilaki M, et al: Analysis of immunohistochemical results of the *ras* oncogene product p21 in myelodysplastic syndromes. *Anticancer Res* 13:1103–1106, 1993.

Kroef MJ, Bolk MW, Willemze, et al: Absence of loss of heterozygosity of the *IRF1* gene in some patients with 5q31 deletion. *Blood* 83:2382, 1994.

Liu E, Hjelle B, Morgan R, et al: Mutations of the *Kirsten-ras* proto-oncogene in human preleukemia. *Nature* 330:186–188, 1987.

Ludwig L, Schulz AS, Janssen JW, et al: p53 Mutations in myelodysplastic syndromes. *Leukemia* 6:1302–1304, 1992.

Lyons J, Janssen JWG, Bartram C, et al: Mutation of Ki-*ras* and N-*ras* oncogenes in myelodysplastic syndromes. *Blood* 71:1707–1712, 1988.

Marsh JCW, Geary CG: Is aplastic anaemia a pre-leukaemic disorder? *Br J Haematol* 77:447–452, 1991.

Marshall CJ: How does p21 ras transform cells? *Trends Genet* 7:91–95, 1991a.

Marshall CJ: Tumor suppressor genes: *Cell* 64:313–326, 1991b.

Melani C, Haliassos A, Chomel JC, et al: Ras activation in myelodysplastic syndromes: Clinical and molecular study of the chronic phase of the disease. *Br J Haemotol* 74:408–413, 1990.

Miyake K, Inokuchi K, Dan K, et al: Alterations in the deleted colorectal carcinoma gene in human primary leukemia. *Blood* 82:927–930, 1993a.

Miyake K, Inokuchi K, Dan K, et al: Expression of the *DCC* gene in myelodysplastic syndromes and overt leukemia. *Leuk Res* 17:785–788, 1993b.

Needleman SW, Kraus MH, Srivastava SK, et al: High frequency of N-*ras* activation in acute myelogenous leukemia. *Blood* 67:753–757, 1986.

Nimer SD, Golde DW: The 5q-abnormality. *Blood* 70:1705–1712, 1987.

Nowell P, Wilmoth D, Lange B: Cytogenetics of childhood preleukemia. *Cancer Genet Cytogenet* 6:261–266, 1983.

Padua RA, Carter G, Hughes D, et al: RAS mutations in myelodysplasia detected by amplification, oligonucleotide hybridization, and transformation. *Leukemia* 2:503–510, 1988.

Paquette RL, Landaw EM, Pierre RV, et al: N-*ras* mutations are associated with poor prognosis and increased risk of leukemia in myelodysplastic syndrome. *Blood* 82:590–599, 1993.

Porfiri E, Secker-Walker LM, Hoffbrand AV, et al: *DCC* tumor suppressor gene is inactivated in hematologic malignancies showing monosomy 18. *Blood* 81:2696–2701, 1993.

Saltman DL, Dolganov GM, Warrington JA, et al: A physical map of 15 loci on human chromosome 5q23–q33 by two color fluorescence in situ hybridization. *Genomics* 16:726–732, 1993.

Sawyers CL, Denny CT: Chronic myelomonocytic leukemia: Tel-a-kinase what Ets all about. *Cell* 77:171–173, 1994.

Shannon KM, O'Connell P, Martin GA, et al: Loss of the normal *NF1* allele from the bone marrow of children with type 1 neurofibromatosis and malignant myeloid disorders. No diagnostic abnormality. *N Engl J Med* 330:597–601, 1994.

Shannon KM, Watterson J, Johnson P, et al: Monosomy 7 myeloproliferative disease in children with neurofibromatosis type 1: Epidemiology and molecular analysis. *Blood* 79:1311–1318, 1992.

Sherr CJ: Colony-stimulating factor-1 receptor. *Blood* 75:1–12, 1990.

Slingerland JM, Minden MD, Benchimol S: Mutation of the p53 gene in human acute myelogenous leukemia. *Blood* 77:1500–1507, 1991.

Springall F, O'Mara S, Shounan Y, et al: *c-fms* Point mutations in acute myeloid leukemia: Fact or fiction? *Leukemia* 7:978–985, 1993.

Sugimoto K, Hirano N, Toyoshima H, et al: Mutations of the p53 gene in myelodysplastic syndrome (MDS) and MDS-derived leukemia. *Blood* 81:3022–3026, 1993.

Tefferi A, Thibodeau SN, Solberg LA Jr: Clonal studies in the myelodysplastic syndrome using X-linked restriction fragment length polymorphisms. *Blood* 75:1770–1773, 1990.

Tsuge I, Kojima S, Matsuoka H, et al: Clonal haematopoiesis in children with acquired aplastic anaemia. *Br J Haematol* 84:137–143, 1993.

van Kamp H, Fibbe WE, Jansen RP, et al: Clonal involvement of granulocytes and monocytes, but not of T and B lymphocytes and natural killer cells, in patients with myelodysplasia: Analysis by X-linked restriction fragment length polymorphisms and polymerase chain reaction of the phosphoglycerate kinase gene. *Blood* 80:1774–1780, 1992.

Van Kamp H, Jansen R, Willemze R, et al: Studies on clonality by PCR analysis of the *PGK*-1 gene. *Nucl Acids Res* 19:2794, 1991.

Vigon I, Dreyfus F, Melle J, et al: Expression of the *c-mpl* proto-oncogene in human hematologic malignancies. *Blood* 82:877–883, 1993.

Vogelstein B, Fearon ER, Hamilton SR, et al: Use of restriction fragment length polymorphisms to determine the clonal origin of human tumors. *Science* 227:642–645, 1985.

Vogelstein B, Fearon ER, Hamilton SR, et al: Clonal analysis using recombinant DNA probes from X-chromosome. *Cancer Res* 47:4806–4813, 1987.

Willman CL, Sever CE, Pallavicini MG, et al: Deletion of *IRF*-1, mapping to chromosome 5q31.1, in human leukemia and preleukemic myelodysplasia. *Science* 259:968–971, 1993.

Yunis JJ, Boot AJM, Mayer MG, et al: Mechanisms of ras mutations in myelodysplastic syndrome. *Oncogene* 4:609–614, 1989.

Yunis JJ, Lobell M, Arnesen MA, et al: Refined chromosome study helps define prognostic subgroups in most patients with primary myelodysplastic syndrome and acute myelogenous leukaemia. *Br J Hematol* 68:189–194, 1988.

Zhang K, DeClue JE, Vass WC, et al: Suppression of *c-ras* transformation by GTPase-activating protein. *Nature* 346:754–756, 1990.

Review Articles: Molecular Genetics

Bartram CR: Molecular genetic aspects of myelodysplastic syndromes. *Hematol Oncol Clin North Am* 6:557–570, 1992.

Bartram CR, Janssen JWG: Oncogenes as diagnostic markers of therapeutic effectiveness in human myeloid leukemias. In Bannaseh P (ed): *Cancer Therapy: Contributions to Oncology,* Vol. 39. Basel, Karger, 1990, pp 169–179.

Carter G, Ridge S, Padua RA: Genetic lesions in preleukemia. *Crit Rev Oncog* 3:339–364, 1992.

Jacobs A, Padua RA, Carter G, et al: *ras* Mutations in the myelodysplastic syndromes. In Schmalzl F, Mufti GJ (eds): *Myelodysplastic Syndromes.* New York, Springer-Verlag, 1992, pp 187–192.

Kreipe HH: Histopathology and molecular pathology of chronic myeloproliferative disorder. *Veroff Pathol* 141:1–158, 1993.

Layton DM: The molecular biology of myelodysplastic syndromes (preleukaemia). In Mufti GJ, Galton DAG (eds): *The Myelodysplastic Syndromes.* New York, Churchill Livingstone, 1992, pp 151–195.

Layton DM, Bartram CR: *ras* Oncogenes in myelodysplastic syndromes. In Schmalzl F, Mufti GJ (eds): *Myelodysplastic Syndromes.* New York, Springer-Verlag, 1992, pp 201–214.

Noel P, Solberg LA Jr: Myelodysplastic syndromes. Pathogenesis, diagnosis and treatment. *Crit Rev Oncol Hematol* 12:193–215, 1992.

Rodenhuis S: *ras* and human tumors. *Semin Cancer Biol* 3:241–247, 1992.

Articles: Cytokines

Ambrus JL Jr, Pippin J, Joseph A, et al: Identification of a cDNA for a human high-molecular weight B-cell growth factor. *Proc Natl Acad Sci USA* 90:6330–6334, 1993.

Barut BA, Cochran MK, O'Hara C, et al: Response patterns of hairy cell leukemia to B-cell mitogens and growth factors. *Blood* 76:2091–2097, 1990.

Brantschen S, de Weck AL, Stadler BM: Factors influencing proliferation and histamine content of cultured human bone marrow cells. *Immunobiology* 179:271–282, 1989.

Brodsky I, Hubbel HR, Strayer DR, et al: Implications of retroviral and oncogene activity in chronic myelogenous leukemia. *Cancer Genet Cytogenet* 26:15–23, 1987.

Dadmarz R, Rabinowe SN, Cannistra SA, et al: Association between clonogenic cell growth and clinical risk group in B-cell chronic lymphocytic leukemia. *Blood* 76:142–149, 1990.

de Vries JE: Novel fundamental approaches to intervening in IgE-mediated allergic diseases. *J Invest Dermatol* 102:141–144, 1994.

Doherty TM, Kastelein R, Menon S, et al: Modulation of murine macrophage function by IL-13. *J Immunol* 151:7151–7160, 1993.

Everson MP, Brown CB, Lilly MB: Interleukin-6 and granulocyte-macrophage colony-stimulating factor are candidate growth factors for chronic myelomonocytic leukemia cells. *Blood* 74:1472–1476, 1989.

Grabstein KH, Eisenman J, Shanebeck K, et al: Cloning of a T cell growth factor that interacts with the B chain of the interleukin-2 receptor. *Science* 264:965–968, 1994.

Hounsell J, Isbister JP: What's new in haematology? *Med J Aust* 160:38–40, 1994.

Kiniwa M, Gately M, Gubler U, et al: Recombinant interleukin-12 suppresses the synthesis of immunoglobulin E by interleukin-4 stimulated human lymphocytes. *J Clin Invest* 90:262–270, 1992.

Lee F, Yokota T, Otsuka T, et al: Isolation and characterization of a mouse interleukin cDNA clone that expresses B-cell stimulatory factor 1 activities and T-cell- and mast-cell-stimulating activities. *Proc Natl Acad Sci USA* 83:2061–2065, 1986.

Lin FK, Suggs S, Lin CH, et al: Cloning and expression of the human erythropoietin gene. *Proc Natl Acad Sci USA* 82:7580–7584, 1985.

Maurer AB, Gansu A, Buhl R, et al: Restoration of impaired cytokine secretion from monocytes of patients with myelodysplastic syndromes after in vivo treatment with GM-CSF or IL-3. *Leukemia* 7:1728–1733, 1993.

Nagata S, Tsuchiya M, Asano S, et al: Molecular cloning and expression of cDNA for human granulocyte colony stimulating factor. *Nature* 319:415–418, 1986.

Newcom SR, Kadin ME, Ansari AA: Production of transforming growth factor-beta activity by Ki-1 positive lymphoma cells and analysis of its role in the regulation of Ki-1 positive lymphoma growth. *Am J Pathol* 131:569–577, 1988.

Nickoloff BJ, Mitra RS, Elder JT, et al: Decreased growth inhibition by recombinant gamma interferon is associated with increased transforming growth factor-alpha production in keratinocytes cultured from psoriatic lesions. *Br J Dermatol* 121:161–174, 1989.

Nimer SD, Gasson JC, Hu K, et al: Activation of the GM-CSF promoter by HTLV-I and -II tax proteins. *Oncogene* 4:671–676, 1989.

Punnonen J, de Vries JE: IL-13 induces proliferation, Ig isotype switching, and Ig synthesis by immature human fetal B cells. *J Immunol* 152:1094–1102, 1994.

Razzano M, Coslini C, Cortelazzo S, et al: Clinical and biological effects of erythropoietin treatment of myelodysplastic syndrome. *Leuk-Lymphoma* 10:127–134, 1993.

Ridge SA, Worwood M, Oscier D, et al: FMS mutations in myelodysplastic, leukemic, and normal subjects. *Proc Natl Acad Sci USA* 87:1377–1380, 1990.

Sanderson CJ, O'Garra A, Warren DJ, et al: Eosinophil differentiation factor also has B-cell growth factor activity: Proposed name interleukin 4. *Proc Natl Acad Sci USA* 83:437–440, 1986.

Sporn MB, Roberts AB: Autocrine growth factors and cancer. *Nature* 313:745–747, 1985.

Uckun FM, Fauci AS, Chandan-Langlie M, et al: Detection and characterization of human high molecular weight B cell growth factor receptors on leukemic B cells in chronic lymphocytic leukemia. *J Clin Invest* 84:1595–1608, 1989.

Wakasugi N, Tagaya Y, Wakasugi H, et al: Adult T-cell leukemia derived factor/thioredoxin, produced by both human T-lymphotropic virus type I and Epstein-Barr virus transformed lymphocytes, acts as an autocrine growth factor and synergizes with interleukin 1 and interleukin 2. *Proc Natl Acad Sci USA* 87:8282–8286, 1990.

Wang Z, Gao XZ, Preisler HD: Studies of the proliferation and differentiation of immature myeloid cells in vitro: I. Chronic myelogenous leukemia. *Am J Hematol* 30:77–81, 1989.

Wong GG, Temple PA, Leary AC, et al: Human CSF-1: Molecular cloning and expression of 4-kb cDNA encoding the human urinary protein. *Science* 235:1504–1508, 1987.

Wong GG, Witek-Giannotti JS, Temple PA, et al: Stimulation of murine hemopoietic colony formation by human IL-6. *J Immunol* 140:3040–3044, 1988.

Woods GM, Sawyer PJ, Kirov SM, et al: Functional and phenotypic analysis of a T cell prolymphocytic leukemia. *Leuk Res* 9:587–596, 1985.

Yang YC, Ciarletta AB, Temple PA, et al: Human IL-3 (multi-CSF): Identification by expression cloning of a novel hematopoietic growth factor related to murine IL-3. *Cell* 47:3–10, 1986.

Review Articles: Cytokines

Aggarwal BB, Gutterman JU: *Human Cytokines: Handbook for Basic and Clinical Research*. Boston, Blackwell Scientific, 1992.

Andreeff M, Welte K: Hematopoietic colony stimulating factors. *Semin Oncol* 16:211–229, 1989.

Chiu IM: Growth factor genes as oncogenes. *Mol Chem Neuropathol* 10:37–52, 1989.

Clark SC, Kamen R: The human hematopoietic colony-stimulating factors. *Science* 236:1229–1237, 1987.

Costello RT: Therapeutic use of granulocyte-macrophage colony-stimulating factor (GM-CSF). A review of recent experience. *Acta Oncol* 32:403–408, 1993.

Demetri GD, Griffin JD: Hemopoietins and leukemia. *Hematol Oncol Clin North Am* 3:535–553, 1989.

Friedman WH, Michon J: Pathophysiology of cytokines. *Leuk Res* 14:675–677, 1990.

Goldstone AH, Khwaja A: The role of haemopoietic growth factors in bone marrow transplantation. *Leuk Res* 14:721–729, 1990.

Gutterman JU: Cytokine therapeutics: Lessons from interferon alpha. *Proc Natl Acad Sci USA* 91:1198–1205, 1994.

Holmlund JT: Cytokines. *Cancer Chemother Biol Response Modif* 14:150–206, 1993.

Kawano M, Kuramoto A, Hirano T, et al: Cytokines as autocrine growth factors in malignancies. *Cancer Surv* 8:905–919, 1989.

Kelleher K, Bean K, Clark SC, et al: Human interleukin-9: Genomic sequence, chromosomal location, and sequences essential for its expression in human T-cell leukemia virus (HTLV)-1-transformed human T cells. *Blood* 77:1436–1441, 1991.

Lang RA, Burgess AW: Autocrine growth factors and tumorigenic transformation. *Immunol Today* 11:244–249, 1990.

Lee F: Growth factors controlling the development of hemopoietic cells. *Prog Clin Biol Res* 352:385–390, 1990.

Leonard EJ, Yoshimura T: Human monocyte chemoattractant protein-1 (MCP-1). *Immunol Today* 11:97–101, 1990.

Metcalf D: Haemopoietic growth factors 2: Clinical applications. *Lancet* 1:885–887, 1989a.

Mecalf D: The molecular control of cell division, differentiation, commitment and maturation in haemopoietic cells. *Nature* 339:27–30, 1989b.

Moore MA: Hematopoietic growth factors in cancer. *Cancer* 65:836–844, 1990.

Neidhart JA: Hematopoietic cytokines. Current use in cancer therapy. *Cancer* 72(Suppl 11):3381–3386, 1993.

Olsson I, Olofsson T: Tumor associated myelopoiesis inhibiting factors. *Leuk Res* 14:715–716, 1990.

Paul SR, Bennett F, Calvetti JA, et al: Molecular cloning of a cDNA encoding interleukin 11, a stromal cell-derived lymphopoietic and hematopoietic cytokine. *Proc Natl Acad Sci USA* 87:7512–7516, 1990.

Paul SR, Yang YC, Donahue RE, et al: Stromal cell-associated hematopoiesis: Immortalization and characterization of a primate bone marrow-derived stromal cell line. *Blood* 77:1723–1733, 1991.

Quesenberry P, Souza L, Krantz S: *Growth Factors. Education Program.* Atlanta, Georgia American Society of Hematology, 1989, pp 98–113.

Raso V: Growth factors and other ligands. *Cancer Treat Res* 37:297–320, 1988.

Robertson MJ, Ritz J: Biology and clinical relevance of human natural killer cells. *Blood* 76:2421–2438, 1990.

Schottner A: Lymphokines in autoimmunity: A critical review. *Clin Immunol Immunopathol* 70:177–189, 1994.

Schuster MW: Will cytokines alter the treatment of myelodysplastic syndrome? *Am J Med Sci* 305:72–78, 1993.

Testa NG, Dexter TM: Haemopoietic growth factors and hematological malignancies. *Baillieres Clin Endocrinol Metab* 4:177–189, 1990.

Thompson-Snipes L, Dhar V, Bond MW, et al: Interleukin 10: A novel stimulatory factor for mast cells and their progenitors. *J Exp Med* 173:507–510, 1991.

Touw I, Pouwels K, van Agthoven T, et al: Interleukin-7 is a growth factor of precursor B and T acute lymphoblastic leukemia. *Blood* 75:2097–2101, 1990.

Vieira P, de Waal-Malefyt R, Dang MN, et al: Isolation and expression of human cytokine synthesis inhibitory factor cDNA clones: Homology to Epstein-Barr virus open reading frame BCRFI. *Proc Natl Acad Sci USA* 88:1172–1176, 1991.

CHAPTER **9**

Clinical Features, Prognosis, and Treatment

CLINICAL FEATURES

Incidence, Symptoms, and Signs

There are no precise data on the incidence of MDSs. In 1983, there were 579 new cases of MDSs in France. In the United States, it is estimated that there are about 1,500 new cases per year. Population-based estimates in Dusseldorf indicate that the annual incidence of MDSs is about 4.1/100,000. Between the ages of 50 and 70 years the incidence was 4.9/100,000, but in patients over the age of 70 it escalated to 22.8/100,000. (Fig. 9.1)

MDSs primarily affect the elderly, though it can be seen at any age. Most studies indicate a peak incidence in the eighth decade of life. The median age in one survey was 72 years, with only 6.7% of patients being younger than 50 and 83.9% being over 60. The incidence appears to have increased over the last 20 years, though this may be partly due to an increased awareness of the MDSs. Females are affected about 1.5 times more frequently than males. At presentation, about 21% have RA, 24% have RARS, 23% have RAEB, 16% have RAEB-IT, and about 16% have CMML. These percentages vary in different series.

The presenting symptoms of MDS are usually nonspecific, and some patients are diagnosed accidentally when a complete blood count (CBC) is performed for unrelated reasons. However, up to 90% of patients are symptomatic at the time of diagnosis. The most common symptoms are fatigue (87%), weight loss (29%), bleeding (24%), and fever (24%). Weight loss may be more severe in patients with

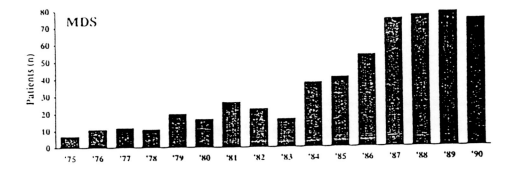

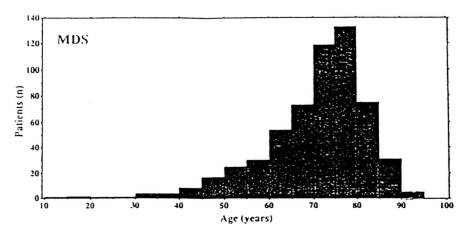

Figure 9.1   Annual incidence of MDSs in the Dusseldorf Bone Marrow Registry (top) and age distribution of these cases. (Adapted from Aul C, Gatterman N, Schneider W: Age related incidence and other epidemiological aspects of myelodysplastic syndromes. *Br J Haematol* 82:358–367, 1992.

CMML, while bleeding and fever are more common in patients with RAEB and RAEB-IT. Physical examination may reveal petechiae/purpura (26%), splenomegaly (17%), and hepatomegaly (12%). Eventually, sepsis accounts for about 40% and bleeding complications for about 21% of the deaths in MDS. At times, the MDSs may present in an unusual fashion or may be associated with another disorder. Patients with MDSs have been reported to present with cutaneous granulocytic sarcomas. Vasculitis, gamma heavy chain disease, Crohn's disease, and solid tumors have been reported to occur in association with MDSs. According to one report, there may be a higher risk of MDSs in the families of patients with these disorders.

MDSs occasionally occur in pregnancy and appear to transform rapidly into acute leukemia in most of these patients. Whether pregnancy affects the leukemogenic potential of the disease is not clear. Primary MDS in children is a rare event; 144 cases have been reported in the pediatric literature through 1992. Regardless of the FAB subtype, pediatric MDSs appear to have an aggressive clinical course. The incidence of leukemic transformation is high, and median survival of the whole group is only 9.9 months.

Laboratory Abnormalities

In addition to the cytopenias and the increase in the monocyte count or blast count (see Chapter 2), MDSs are frequently associated with biochemical and functional abnormalities of neutrophils, erythrocytes, and platelets. The neutrophils may have myeloperoxidase or, in about 20% of the cases, alkaline phosphatase deficiency. Erythrocytes may become deficient in a number of glycolytic enzymes, most frequently pyruvate kinase. About 80% of MDS patients have an increase in fetal hemoglobin synthesis. The stimulus for this increase is not known. About 8% of patients show an increase in hemoglobin H (tetramer of beta globin chains), and this may occur prior to leukemic transformation. Changes in blood group expression have also been seen in patients with MDSs. This has included an increase in the expression of "i" antigen and a decrease in A1 and H substance. About 20% of patients with MDSs exhibit an increase in lysozyme activity in blood and urine. This may reflect increased neutrophil and monocyte turnover. The platelets have decreased adhesion to collagen and have defective aggregation with ADP or collagen. There may be loss of the dense granule storage pool and, rarely, a membrane defect resembling that of Bernard Soulier syndrome. In functional terms, neutrophils in MDSs exhibit decreased adhesion, phagocytosis, and bactericidal activity. The bleeding time, even with a normal platelet count, may be long. There are also reports of a high incidence of hypergammaglobulinemia (32%), a positive direct antiglobulin test (8%), and the presence of other autoantibodies in patients with MDSs. Whether these phenomena are the result of infections and transfusions, or are due to lymphocytic malfunctions in MDSs, is not clear.

Natural History of the MDSs

Because of the heterogeneity of the involved subgroups, their natural history also shows marked variation. In general, RA and RARS follow an indolent course with relatively long survival, but the other three subgroups are aggressive disorders with a much higher incidence of leukemic transformation and short survival. Hence, clinically, one can divide the MDSs into two major groups: the first one consisting of RA and RARS and having a more benign course; and the second group consisting of CMML, RAEB, and RAEB-IT, which are aggressive, have a higher incidence of leukemic transformation, and have a shorter survival.

By obtaining sequential morphological and cytogenetic data in 46 patients over 10 years, Tricot and associates (1985) have suggested that MDS may evolve in four ways:

1. Evolution pattern A, in which the disease remains stable with minimal or no increase in the blast percentage. This is seen in 48% of the cases.
2. Evolution pattern B, in which the disease remains stable for a period of time and then transforms abruptly into acute leukemia. This is seen in about 25% of the cases
3. Evolution pattern C, in which a gradual increase in the blast percentage in the marrow occurs. A majority of these patients eventually develop acute leukemia. This is seen in 24% of the patients.

Table 9.1   Median Survival (in Months) of MDSs by FAB Classification

Author	No. of Patients	RA	RARS	CMML	RAEB	RAEB-IT
Coiffier	193	41	52.5	11.5	14.5	6.5
Vallespi	101	17	16	5	14	2.5
Mufti	141	32	76	22	10.5	5
Varela	60	47	52	15	14	3
Weisdorf	69	52	29	2	12	11
Tricot	85	18.5	21.5	9.5	11	4.5
Todd	326	42	36	17.5	17.5	NA
Foucar	109	64	71	8	7	5
Mean		39.1	44.2	11.3	12.5	5.3

Abbreviations: NA = not available.

4. Evolution pattern D, in which the malignant clone has a marked proliferative capacity. This is typically associated with therapy-related MDS. In this study, acquisition of new cytogenetic lesions was invariably associated with transformation to acute leukemia.

Refractory Anemia with Ringed Sideroblasts (RARS):   Patients with RARS are mostly in their 70s at the time of diagnosis, and the disease is well advanced at the time of presentation. All patients are, as a rule, anemic, and about a third are neutropenic and/or thrombocytopenic. About 70% are or become transfusion dependent. Those who do not require transfusions have the best survival. Once transfusions become necessary, mean survival is 1–3 years. This probably reflects a more severe disease process and the added problem of iron overload due to the transfusions. For the whole group, median survival varies widely among the reported studies (Table 9.1), ranging from 16 to 76 months (mean, 44.25 months). Compared to the other subgroups, the incidence of leukemic transformation is low in this group, ranging from 0% to 19% (Table 9.2). Patients with neutropenia and thrombocytopenia appear to have a higher risk of leukemogenesis.

Refractory Anemia (RA):   The demographic features of the patient population are similar to those of RARS. About 50% of the patients with RA present with a monocytopenia (30% have anemia), about 36% with bicytopenia, and the rest with pancytopenia. The incidence of leukemic transformation ranges from 17% to 21% in the large series. Median survival ranges from 17 to 64 months (mean, 39.1 months).

Table 9.2   Incidence of Leukemic Transformation in Myelodysplastic Syndromes

Author	No. of Patients	RA	RARS (%)	CMML	RAEB	RAEB-IT
Foucar	109	18	0	33	33	44
Todd	326	21	19	34	44	67
Tricot*	418	17	6	16	57	20
Mean		18.6	8.3	27.6	44.6	43.6

*Combined data from three studies.

The 5q− syndrome is a refractory anemia with an interstitial deletion of the long arm of chromosome 5 (q13–q31). Patients with this disorder have macrocytic anemia, thrombocytosis, and nonlobulated megakaryocytes in the bone marrow. The clinical course is benign and protracted, with little risk of leukemic transformation. However, since the original description of this syndrome in 1974 by Van den Berghe et al., deletions of 5q have been described not only in patients with RA, but also in those with RARS, RAEB, and RAEB-IT. If the patient had additional chromosomal abnormalities, the disease was labeled type B 5q− (5q− alone being type A). 5q− has also been described in myeloproliferative disorders, acute leukemia, and even solid tumors, raising doubts about whether the 5q− syndrome is a separate clinical entity. One of the larger series of patients who had MDSs and 5q− was recently published by Mathew et al. (1993) from the Mayo Clinic and included 43 consecutive patients. Of this group, 72% belonged to the RA subgroup, 7% to RARS, 16% to RAEB, and 5% to RAEB-IT. The projected median survival for the whole group was 63 months. The incidence of leukemic transformation was 16% and was uniformly fatal. Patients with RAEB and RAEB-IT did poorly compared to the other FAB subgroups. Therapy, in general, was unsuccessful.

Chronic Myelomonocytic Leukemia (CMML):   The median age at diagnosis of CMML is 66 years, and the male:female ratio is 2.4:1. Development of CMML is preceded by a different type of MDS in about 24% of the cases. Chromosomal abnormalities are seen in about 34% of these patients; trisomy 8, monosomy 7, and deletion of the long arm of chromosome 20 being the more common lesions. The median survival is shorter compared to RA and RARS, ranging from 2.0 to 22 months (mean, 11.3 months). The risk of leukemic transformation is 16–34% (mean, 27.6%).

Refractory Anemia with Excess Blasts (RAEB) and RAEB in Transformation to Acute Leukemia (RAEB-IT):   The age and sex distribution of patients with RAEB than RAEB-IT are similar to those of the other FAB subgroups of MDSs. However, as in CMML, these patients have more severe cytopenias and tend to be sicker due to a higher frequency of febrile and hemorrhagic complications. The evolution of the disease is slower in RAEB than in RAEB-IT, as shown by better survival in the former. In large series, the median survival for RAEB ranged from 7 to 17.5 months (mean, 12.5 months), and for RAEB-IT it was 2.5 to 11 months (mean, 5.3 months). Thus, in RAEB, with close monitoring, one can assess the pace of the disease and tailor the therapy accordingly. In patients with stable blood counts, close monitoring may be sufficient initially. Patients with RAEB-IT, in general, have severe cytopenias and the consequent complications at the time of diagnosis, and are frequently treated as having acute leukemia.

The question of leukemic transformation in RAEB, and especially in RAEB-IT, becomes somewhat moot. The major consequence of these disorders is the cytopenias, and it is the severity of the cytopenias (particularly neutropenia and thrombocytopenia) that determines the therapeutic approach in a given patient. Thus, a patient may have all the clinical problems seen in acute leukemia without meeting the diagnostic criteria of that disorder. In these situations, it is entirely reasonable to treat the patient with acute leukemia therapy.

On the other hand, biological questions posed by RAEB and RAEB-IT remain interesting. As shown by the cytogenetic and morphological markers, the leukemic

Table 9.3   Evolution of Aplastic Anemia into an MDS or Acute Leukemia

Author	No. of Patients	Follow-up (years)	To MDS (%)	To Acute Leukemia (%)
Tichelli	117	14	11	17
de Planque	223	7	11	19

clone has already established itself in the bone marrow. Why does the disease take longer to evolve in RAEB and RAEB-IT? Is this essentially a matter of the absolute number of blasts in the bone marrow, or is the disease biologically different in these two entities? The answers to these questions may be important in devising therapeutic approaches in RAEB and RAEB-IT.

Overall survival for the MDSs is 54% at 1 year, 34% at 2 years, 23% at 3 years, 17% at 4 years, and only 8.3% at 5 years.

Acute Leukemia Following MDSs

There are rare examples of the development of ALL in patients with MDSs. However, in virtually all patients, the transformation is to an AML. The morphological and cytochemical features of these acute leukemias are similar to those of de novo acute leukemias. Most cases of AML which evolve from MDS belong to the M1, M2, M4, and M6 subtypes of the FAB classification. However, acute promyelocytic leukemia (M3) has also been occasionally reported to occur.

The blast cells in acute leukemia evolving from a MDS differ from those evolving from a de novo acute leukemia in certain respects. The former frequently show an expression of the lymphocyte activating antigens CD25 and CD30 on their surfaces. These blasts also do not respond to the suppressive effect of transforming growth factor beta 1 (TGFb1) in vitro. Their lack of response to TGFb1 is due to a decrease in the number of high-affinity receptors for this agent. On the other hand, in vitro growth patterns and the response to various growth factors are very similar in blasts from de novo acute leukemia and those evolving from the MDSs.

Evolution of Aplastic Anemia to MDSs

Early in the 1950s, it was recognized that a small number of cases of aplastic anemia may evolve into MDSs and acute leukemia. Retrospective series report an incidence of 1% to 3% between 1950 and 1970. Similarly, paroxysmal nocturnal hemoglobinuria (PNH), which is a monoclonal preleukemic state and frequently presents with hypoplastic bone marrow, can transform into acute leukemia (Table 9.3).

Over the last few years, it has become clear that in many patients, features of both MDS and aplastic anemia are present. Hypoplastic MDS has been described as a distinct clinicopathological entity. By using RFLPs of the X-linked genes, hematopoiesis in 13 out of 18 (72%) patients with acquired aplastic anemia was found to be clonal. In a study by Tichelli et al. (1992), 117 patients with aplastic anemia were followed over a 14-year period. Eleven developed MDSs, and 17 developed PNH. The authors calculated that the cumulative risk of developing a clonal hematopoietic disorder in aplastic anemia at 10 years is 42%. In a Swiss study of 103 patients with aplastic anemia 13 developed PNH and 8 developed myelodysplastic syndrome or acute leukemia. A European Cooperative Group study has reported on the long-term follow-up of 223 patients with aplastic anemia who were treated with immunosuppressive therapy. They had a 13% risk of developing PNH and a 15% risk of developing either MDS or acute leukemia at 7 years. All these studies demonstrate that in a substantial number of patients, aplastic anemia is associated with a clonal hematopoiesis, which may evolve into PNH and MDS/acute leukemia. It is also important to realize that virtually all these patients were treated with immunosuppressive therapy prior to the development of a clonal disorder. What role immunosuppressive therapy plays in this situation is not clear. Rarely, patients with MDS have been shown to evolve into aplastic anemia.

PROGNOSIS

Numerous studies have tried to identify the prognostic factors in MDSs. The parameters that have been analyzed are the FAB classification, age, sex, hemoglobin level, neutrophil count, platelet count, monocyte count, presence of circulating blasts, presence of hemolysis by chromium 51 labeling, iron uptake by marrow erythroid precursors, dysplastic changes of the bone marrow, surface antigens of the marrow progenitors, percentage of bone marrow blasts, cytogenetic abnormalities of the marrow precursor cells, in vitro growth patterns of the bone marrow, and presence of circulating CD34-positive cells. Most of these data are retrospective.

Garcia et al. (1988) studied 107 patients retrospectively for 37 clinical, biochemical, and hematological parameters and found that the FAB classification was the main prognostic factor for predicting survival. They found that platelet count, hemoglobin level, and circulating erythroblasts were also significantly associated with survival. Coiffier and associates (1983) reported on 193 patients and found that excess bone marrow blasts (more than 5%), neutropenia, thrombocytopenia, and the presence of circulating blasts were, in descending order, most closely associated with survival in MDS. In a long-term prospective study of 326 patients, Todd and Pierre (1986) found that, within each FAB subgroup of MDS, the presence of cytogenetic abnormalities predicted poorer survival. Foucar et al. (1985) reported that FAB classification predicts survival. Tricot et al. (1985) reviewed data from eight studies, with a total number of 851 patients, to determine the prognostic factors in MDS. They considered age, cytopenias, bone marrow histology, cytogenetics, in vitro cultures, iron kinetics, and labeling index of marrow cells. They reported that the percentage of blast cells in the marrow (more vs. less than 5%), the presence of circulating blast cells, and the presence of ALIP predict survival most reliably. Surprisingly, these simple parameters gave more accurate results than more sophisticated ones like cytogenetic abnormalities, in vitro cultures, and labeling index. More recently, a Greek study of 158 patients, also showed that bone marrow blasts are the most important variable in predicting survival in MDS (Table 9.4).

Two studies have reported on prognostic factors in CMML alone. These involved 41 and 107 patients, respectively. In both, the marrow blast count of more than 5% was found to be the most important factor.

Jacobs et al. (1986), in a smaller study of 49 patients, found that the combination

Table 9.4 Prognostic Factors in MDSs

Author	No. of Patients	Study Type	Prognostic Factors Analyzed	Significant Factors
Garcia	107	Retrospective	37 clinical, biochemical, and hematological	FAB, platelet count, Hg
Coiffier	193	Retrospective	Clinical, biochemical, in vitro marrow culture, Fe kinetics	Marrow blasts ≥5%, neutropenia, thrombocytopenia, circulating blasts
Tricot	851	Review of 8 studies	As above, plus cytogenetics	Marrow blasts ≥5%, circulating blasts, ALIP on bone marrow biopsy
Economo-poulos	158	Prospective	Clinical	Marrow blasts ≥5%

of morphology (according to the FAB classification) and cytogenetic abnormalities was the best predictor of survival in MDS.

About half of the patients with MDS have a cytogenetic abnormality. Common cytogenetic abnormalities seen in MDSs include monosomy 7, trisomy 8, loss of the long arm of chromosome 5 (del 5), and loss of chromosome 20 (del 20). More refined techniques of studying bone marrow cytogenetics have improved the sensitivity of this important investigation of patients with MDSs. It is now possible to divide patients into three prognostically significant groups by chromosomal analysis. In the most favorable group, the chromosomal analysis is normal or the patients show 5q−. These patients have a median survival of more than 2 years. The second group, with a median survival of 1–2 years, includes those with trisomy 8. The third group, comprising patients who have complex defects and deletion of chromosome 7, fares the worst, with a median survival of less than 1 year. In a study of 284 consecutive adult patients with MDSs and AML, cytogenetic abnormalities emerged as an independent prognostic factor.

Mutations of the N-*ras* gene are found in a number of human malignancies. In MDS, the frequency of these mutations has been found to be 5–30%. By using PCR amplification and differential oligonucleotide hybridization for the presence of N-*ras* exon I mutations in the bone marrows of 252 patients with MDSs, Paquette and associates (1993) found mutations involving codon 12 in 20 (9%) patients. Individuals with N-*ras* mutations had a significantly higher risk of leukemic transformation and a shorter survival. This mutation remained statistically significant even after stratifying for the bone marrow blast count.

The *FMS* gene encodes the functional cell surface receptor for M-CSF. Point mutations of this gene involving codons 301 and 969 can promote neoplastic transformation. Mutations at codon 301 do so by ligand independence and constitutive tyrosine kinase activity of the receptor; mutations involving codon 969 affect its negative regulatory activity. A study by Ridge et al. (1990) involving 67 patients with MDS and 48 with AML showed that about 13% of the patients had *FMS* mutations. The mutations were more common in patients with CMML and

AML-M4. Fifty-one normal subjects were also studied by these investigators as controls. In one of these normal subjects, *FMS* mutation involving codon 969 was seen in the blood and oral cavity mucosa. The significance of this mutation in apparently healthy persons is not known.

High expression of HLA-DR and low expression of CD11b on the marrow cells in MDSs have been reported to be associated with a high frequency of early leukemic transformation. However, the biological significance of these findings is not clear.

Most of the above data are listed in Table 9.4. Certain concerns arise about drawing any definite conclusions from these studies, since many are retrospective, the number of patients in specific FAB subgroups is variable, and cytogenetic techniques vary from study to study. However, one parameter that has been shown to be consistently significant in a majority of these reports is the percentage of blasts in the bone marrow. It appears that patients with more than 5% blasts in the marrow have a shorter survival than those with a lower blast count.

Hirst and associates (1993) have combined hematological parameters, bone marrow blast count, presence of ALIP, and marrow cytogenetics to place patients with MDS into three prognostically different groups:

1. Low-risk group: Peripheral blood score 1, marrow blasts less than 5%, and cytogenetics normal or showing 5q−.
2. Intermediate-risk group: Peripheral blood score 2, marrow blasts 5–10%, presence of ALIP, simple cytogenetic abnormality or trisomy 8.
3. High risk group: Peripheral blood score 3, marrow blasts more than 10%, and complex cytogenetic lesions or monosomy 7.
   Peripheral blood scores: Hemoglobin, 10 g/dL or less = 1; neutrophil count 2.5×10^9/L or less = 1, platelet count 100×10^9/L or less = 1.

This schema has used the most significant prognostic parameters reported so far, and it can help clinicians assess the prognosis in a given patient. Patients in clinical trials can also be stratified by this approach to compare prognostically similar groups of patients across the FAB boundaries.

The Bournemoth scoring system and the scoring system by Sanz were discussed in Chapter 2. These two systems rely primarily on the clinical data and do not incorporate the cytogenetic abnormalities.

TREATMENT OF MDSs

Since there are marked differences in the clinical features and course of the various subgroups (according to the FAB classification) of the MDSs, no simple guidelines exist to assist the clinician in the management of these cases. Treatment decisions are primarily dictated by the severity of the cytopenias and the blast count in the bone marrow and blood. It is also true that the clinical expression of the disease is dependent on the degree of cytopenias. Thus, one may see a patient who is completely asymptomatic, has been found to be anemic on a routine examination, and is diagnosed to have RARS. In such a patient, observation alone may be sufficient. On the other hand, a patient may present with severe neutropenia, fever, thrombocytopenia with bleeding, and 23% blasts in the bone marrow. This patient will have the diagnosis of RAEB-IT. It will be reasonable to treat this patient as having an acute leukemia, as he or she presents with all the complications seen in that disease. Therefore, treatment of a patient with MDS has to be tailored individually.

The treatment modalities available for MDSs can be classified into the following groups:

1. Supportive care
2. B vitamins, corticosteroids, and androgens
3. Differentiation-inducing agents
4. Hematopoietic growth factors and biological response modifiers
5. Chemotherapy
6. Bone marrow transplantation

Supportive Care

This approach includes close observation of the patient, maintenance of a safe hemoglobin level, and management of complications resulting from neutropenia and thrombocytopenia. Patients who develop mild neutropenia and thrombocytopenia can be watched but may need prophylactic antibiotic therapy or platelet transfusions for invasive procedures or surgery. With improvement in the home delivery of health care, it is frequently possible to transfuse patients at home or in the outpatient clinic. Patients who have an absolute neutrophil count of less than 0.5×10^9/L are at great risk of serious or even fatal infections. A temperature of 101°F in such patients should be treated with intravenous antibiotics in the hospital. A platelet count of less than 10×10^9/L is frequently associated with serious bleeding. Platelet transfusions may become necessary in some patients. Agents like epsilon aminocaproic acid should be used as adjunctive therapy in severely thrombocytopenic patients with bleeding complications.

The transfusion of packed red cells and platelets exposes the patient to the usual acute and delayed complications of blood component therapy. In patients requiring regular packed red cell infusions, iron overload becomes an important issue. An average packed red cell unit has about 200 mg of iron. Most of this iron is retained, as it is poorly excreted by the body. Transfusion of 100 packed red cell units will give an overload of 20 g, at which time most adults start to exhibit signs and symptoms of hemochromatosis. These include darkening (graying) of the skin color and the development of diabetes, cardiac arrhythmia, congestive heart failure, and various endocrine abnormalities due to iron deposition in the pituitary. The development of congestive heart failure is an ominous sign, as patients have a short survival after it occurs. The treatment of iron overload is difficult. At present, the only agent available in the United States is deferoxamine, which has to be given parenterally with a pump, is costly, and has significant toxicity. Oral iron chelators are currently being investigated for their safety and efficacy.

After repeated platelet transfusions, about 75% of the patients become refractory because of the development of alloantibodies directed primarily toward the HLA antigens. Use of single-donor platelets or HLA-matched platelets may become necessary in some situations. Infusion of intravenous gammaglobulin prior to the platelet transfusion may enhance platelet survival. Agents like aminocaproic acid may be helpful in the management of such patients.

B Vitamins, Corticosteroids, and Androgens

Since the early 1970s, pyridoxine, in doses of 50–120 mg/day, has been tried in patients with RARS. This was based on the observation that these patients had reduced pyridoxal kinase activity in their red cells and low blood levels of pyridoxal sulfate. However, most patients did not respond to this therapy. There is no known beneficial effect of pyridoxine in other subgroups of the MDSs. Folic acid has also been used empirically in these patients, sometimes with pyridoxine, but has no known benefit.

The reported clinical experience with corticosteroids in MDSs is minimal. Bagby and Gabourel (1980) cultured bone marrows of 54 patients with MDSs in the presence and absence of cortisol. Thirty-four of these patients were treated with oral prednisone in doses that varied between 20 and 160 mg/day. Bone marrows of 29 of these patients failed to show enhanced in vitro growth with cortisone, and none of these patients responded to prednisone. Three of the five patients whose marrow responded to cortisone in culture responded to oral prednisone and showed improvement in their blood counts. Four of these five patients developed acute leukemia 3.5 to 29 months after starting prednisone therapy. More recently, Motoji and colleagues (1990) reported on the use of high-dose methylprednisolone in patients with MDSs. Two of the five patients with RA responded, but none of the six patients with RAEB showed any improvement. Thus, corticosteroids may benefit an occasional patient with MDS but in general appear to have little role in its management. Since a majority of patients do not show in vitro improvement, a screening process to determine the potential benefit of corticoids seems unjustified. The effect of corticoids on the risk of leukemic transformation is not known.

Danazol, a synthetic attenuated androgen, is useful in the management of idiopathic thrombocytopenic purpura. It down-regulates the Fc gamma receptors on monocytes, thereby decreasing the capture of antibody-coated platelets. It has been tried in a selected population of 25 patients with MDS, a majority of whom had elevated levels of platelet-associated IgG. Thirteen of these patients showed improvement in their platelet counts. There was no remarkable effect on the hematopoiesis. These results appear to be similar to those seen in idiopathic thrombocytopenic purpura. Therefore, it appears that danazol has no effect on the myelodysplasia, but it improves platelet survival by decreasing the number of monocyte Fc gamma receptors. Its use should be considered in patients with MDS with significant thrombocytopenia who also show high levels of platelet-associated antibodies.

Differentiation-Inducing Agents

Since maturation block is a feature of myelodysplasia as well as of acute leukemia, agents that induce differentiation in the hematopoietic precursors have always fascinated physicians interested in these disorders. Over the last three decades, many agents have been tried in vitro to promote maturation in various cell lines or marrow cultures of patients. Some of these agents were found to be promising and safe enough to be tried in patients. These include retinoids, vitamin D analogs, hexamethylene bisacetamide, and 5 azacytidine.

Retinoids: Vitamin A and its analogs are necessary for the growth and maturation of normal tissues. They exert their effects by modulating the transcription of genes critical for cellular differentiation. This is carried out by binding of the retinoids to the nuclear retinoic acid receptors, which act as ligand-inducible factors that regulate gene transcription. Cis- and all trans-retinoic acids are the two naturally occurring isomers of retinoic acid. In vitro studies show that both cis- and trans-retinoic acid are capable of inducing differentiation in various leukemia cell lines. In some studies, trans-retinoic acid did this at a concentration which was one log lower than that of the cis-retinoic acid. Retinoids have been found to be clinically useful in a variety of premalignant and malignant conditions such as leukoplakia of the oral cavity, basal cell carcinoma, squamous cell carcinoma of the skin, and T-cell lymphoma of the skin. Retinoids can decrease the risk of a second malignancy of the upper aerodigestive tract in patients with head and neck cancer. Their most dramatic effect is in acute promyelocytic leukemia, in which virtually all patients have a 15:17 translocation. The breakpoint at chromosome 17 involves the gene for the retinoic acid receptor alpha. All trans-retinoic acid can induce clonal remissions in a majority of the patients with acute promyelocytic leukemia, even though its mechanism of action is not clear.

The experience with retinoids in MDSs is fairly extensive. There are nine different studies on the use of cis-retinoic acid in myelodysplasia. A total of 153 patients were treated with doses that ranged between 20 mg/m^2/day to 125 mg/m^2/day for 4–30 weeks. When the data from these studies are combined, it appears that about 20% of patients experienced improvement in their blood counts. Though one of the randomized studies, by Clarke and associates (1987), showed a survival benefit for patients treated with cis-retinoic acid, subsequent randomized studies failed to confirm this finding. In some of these studies, no beneficial effect of cis-retinoic acid could be demonstrated. In 1993, there were two studies on the use of all trans-retinoic acids in MDSs. A total of 62 patients received doses ranging from 10 to 250 mg/m^2/day. Minimal improvements in blood count were seen in four patients, suggesting that all trans-retinoic acid was not a useful agent in MDSs.

Toxicity seen with retinoids includes cheilosis, mucositis, dermatitis, nausea, lethargy, sensorineural hearing loss, headache, and hypertriglyceridemia. The most significant, and dose-limiting, toxicity is hepatoxicity. This is manifested by elevation of transaminase levels and hyperbilirubinemia. Liver functions should be monitored regularly in these patients.

At present, evidence supporting the use of cis-retinoic acids in MDSs is weak. They improve blood counts in a small number of patients but do not appear to have an impact on survival. Because they are relatively nontoxic, their use can be considered in patients who have an indolent form of disease. However, based on the data available so far, all-trans retinoic acid is ineffective in myelodysplasia, and its use is not recommended (Table 9.5).

1,25: Dihydroxyvitamin D$_3$:   This is the biologically active metabolite of vitamin D$_3$ and is a major hormonal regulator of calcium metabolism. More recent studies show that 1,25 dihydroxyvitamin D$_3$ can also induce differentiation in leukemic

Table 9.5 Larger Trials of Retinoic Acid Analogs in MDSs

Author	No. of Patients	Dose and Duration of Treatment	(CR + PR)
		Cis-Retinoic Acid	
Gold	15	20–125 mg/m^2/day for 7–30 wks	33%
Greenberg	18	1–2 mg/kg/day for >8 wks	17%
Swanson	10	2.5–4 mg/kg/day for 8 wks	30%
Picozzi	15	2.5–4 mg/kg/day for 8 wks	33%
Clarke	33	20 mg/m^2/day for 8 wks	9%
Koeffler	35	100 mg/m^2/day for 6 wks	9%
Leoni	20	50–100 mg/m^2/day for >4 wks	60%
		All-Trans-Retinoic Acid	
Kurzrock	39	10–250 mg/m^2/day for 6 wks	3%
Ohno	23	45 mg/m^2/day for 4–16 wks	24%

Abbreviations: CR = complete response; PR = partial response.

cell lines. The clinical experience with this agent, compared to the retinoids, has not been extensive. In three separate reports, 6, 7, and 18 patients were treated with 1,25 dihydroxyvitamin D_3 in doses of 1–2.5 mg/day. Only in the last study (Koeffler et al., 1988) were any responses seen. Seven patients showed minor improvements in blood counts, and one had a 50% increase in platelet, granulocyte, and monocyte counts for 5 weeks. Six patients in this study progressed to acute leukemia.

Side effects of 1,25 dihydroxyvitamin D_3 include nausea, loss of appetite, lethargy, hypercalcemia, polyuria, and polydypsia.

Two other analogs of 1,25 dihydroxyvitamin D_3—24-homo-1,25 dihydroxyvitamin D_3 and 22-oxa-1,25 dihydroxyvitamin D_3—are also being investigated. Neither of these agents has much effect on calcium metabolism. The latter appears to be a much more potent differentiating agent.

Hexamethylene Bisacetamide (HMBA): HMBA is a low molecular weight polar planar compound that has shown significant differentiating activity in the HL-60 and Friend MEL leukemia cell lines. However, the concentrations necessary for differentiation also have been found to be capable of suppressing the growth of committed hematopoietic precursors of normal subjects. Clinical trials to determine the efficacy of HMBA are currently underway. In a study of 41 patients with MDSs, HMBA, given as 5- to 10-day infusions, induced a complete response in three patients and a partial response in six patients. The median duration of the complete response was 6.8 months, and that of the partial response was 3.7 months. The main toxicity of HMBA was thrombocytopenia, which was reversible.

5 Azacytidine: This is an analog of cytidine that incorporates itself in the newly synthesized DNA. It has been tried in acute leukemia, primarily as a second- or third-line therapy, and induces remissions in about 20% of cases. In lower concentrations, 5-azacytidine decreases the activity of DNA methyltransferase, thereby decreasing the methylation of newly synthesized DNA. This hypomethylation is known to alter gene expression. In vitro studies show that lower concentrations of 5-azacytidine can cause differentiation in HL-60 cells. In a study of 11 patients with AML, 5 azacytidine, as a continuous infusion of 75 mg/m²/day, did not produce any responses. In another study of 44 patients with the diagnosis of RAEB or RAEB-IT, the same dose of 5-azacytidine yielded a response rate of 48%, with a complete hematological response in 11% and improvement in blood counts in an additional 37% of the cases. These results are encouraging but need to be confirmed.

Some investigators believe that the effect of low-dose 5 azacytidine, like that of low-dose cytarabine, may be due to its myelotoxic effects rather than its differentiating capabilities. Resolution of this controversy will require further investigation.

Combinations of Differentiating Agents: More recently, combinations of various differentiating agents have been tried in MDSs. In one study, 47 patients with MDSs were treated with interferon alpha in a dose of 3 million U/m²/day, 13 cis-retinoic acid 1 mg/kg/day, and 1,25 dihydoxyvitamin D₃ 1 µg/day. Four patients achieved a complete hematological remission, and nine showed improved blood counts. However, this regimen was quite toxic, with most of the toxicity resulting from the interferon. In another phase II trial, 14 patients were treated with low-dose cytosine arabinoside (5 mg/m² subcutaneously every 12 hr) plus oral cis-retinoic acid, 60 mg/m²/day. Two patients showed improved blood counts. These two trials do not show any survival benefit from combination therapy.

In summary, the differentiating agents are an interesting group of compounds for the treatment of MDS. Cis-retinoic acid, 1,25 dihydroxyvitamin D₃, HMBA, and low-dose 5 azacytidine improve blood counts in a small number of patients over short intervals. All trans-retinoic acid appear ineffective, and combinations of various differentiating agents do not appear to offer any additional advantage. There is no evidence of improvement in survival with single- or multiple-agent therapy. The clinical experience with differentiating agents, with the exception of cis-retinoic acid, is limited, and further investigations will be necessary to determine their role in myelodysplasia.

Hematopoietic Growth Factors and Biological Response Modifiers

Colony-Stimulating Factors: Ever since recombinant colony-stimulating factors became available for clinical trials, they have been tried in MDSs to alleviate the cytopenias. Their use also has been attended by the fear of stimulating the leukemic clone and hastening the development of overt acute leukemia. There is now sufficient clinical experience with erythropoietin, granulocyte-macrophage colony-stimulating factor (GM-CSF), and granulocyte colony-stimulating factor (G-CSF). Early studies with IL-3, and combinations of various colony-stimulating factors have also been completed.

Erythropoietin: Recombinant human erythropoietin is an effective and safe agent in erythropoietin deficiency states such as renal failure. Even though erythropoietin deficiency is not the cause of anemia in myelodysplasia, its use has been justified to stimulate the marrow by pharmacological doses to improve hemoglobin levels and obviate the need for red cell transfusions. It is also true that in a significant percentage of patients with MDSs, erythropoietin levels are inappropriately low.

The largest clinical trial to determine the effect of recombinant erythropoietin in the MDSs was performed by Lessin and associates (1991). In this open-label, randomized, multicenter trial, 177 patients were entered. Erythropoietin was started at 150 U/kg, subcutaneously three times a week, and the dose was escalated. The response was assessed in 100 patients; 28% responded with either a rise of 6% or more in hematocrit values or a decrease in the packed red cell transfusion requirement by 50% or more. The responders had a lower pre-treatment erythropoietin level (32.6–91.3 mU/mL) compared to the nonresponders (168.1 mU/mL). There was minimal toxicity from the treatment. No patient developed seizures, hypertension, or thrombotic disorders. Eight patients developed splenomegaly, presumably from extramedullary hematopoiesis. Five patients progressed to acute leukemia, but the leukemic transformation did not appear to be related to erythropoietin therapy.

The data from other clinical trials of erythropoietin in MDSs can be summarized as follows. A total of 217 patients in 12 different studies were treated with recombinant erythropoietin. In 13% of the patients the hemoglobin level increased, and in an additional 18% there was a decreased need for packed red cell transfusions.

Thus, about 30% of patients with MDSs respond to erythropoietin therapy. The responses are primarily limited to patients with pretherapy serum erythropoietin levels of less than 100 mU/mL. The responses are meaningful in about 18% of the patients, in whom it can reduce the red cell transfusion requirement. Hence, in patients with MDSs with significant or symptomatic anemia, erythropoietin levels should be obtained. If serum levels are less than 100 mU/mL, erythropoietin therapy should be tried.

GM-CSF and G-CSF: GM-CSF is a 20,000-dalton glycoprotein secreted by activated T lymphocytes, endothelial cells, and fibroblasts. It stimulates committed precursors of the granulocytic and macrophage lineages and, to some extent, also promotes pluripotent progenitors to form colonies of erythroid and megakaryocytic cells. G-CSF, a glycoprotein of 19,600 daltons, is normally secreted by monocytes, endothelial cells, and fibroblasts. It stimulates the growth of cells committed to granulocytic differentiation. Recombinant forms of both GM-CSF and G-CSF have been available for clinical trials for many years, and the clinical experience with both agents is fairly extensive.

Between 1987 and 1989, there were five studies on the use of GM-CSF in MDSs. A total of 45 patients were treated in these trials with doses that ranged between 30 and 750 μg/m²/day. Thirty-eight showed improvement in the granulocyte count, 14 had in the reticulocyte count, and 8 in the platelet count. About 10–15% of the patients showed disease progression by an increase in the bone marrow and peripheral blood blast cell counts. These studies prompted the multicenter randomized (treatment with GM-CSF vs. observation) trial in which 133 patients were entered. This large study confirmed the earlier finding that the granulocyte count improved in the vast majority of patients with myelodysplasia treated with GM-CSF, and it translated into fewer infections in these patients. There was, however, no improvement in the hemoglobin level, transfusion requirement, or platelet count. There was also no apparent risk of a higher rate of leukemic transformation with GM-CSF.

The experience with G-CSF is very similar to that with GM-CSF. Fifty-nine patients with MDSs in four different studies were treated with doses that varied from 1 to 5 μg/kg/day. Combined data from these trials showed that 89% of the

Table 9.6   Hematological Response to Recombinant CSFs in MDSs

	GM-CSF	G-CSF	IL-3
No. of patients	45	59	22
Daily dose	30–750 µg/m^2	1–5 µg/kg	30–1000 µg/kg
Response (Increase)			
Neutrophil count	84%	89%	55%
Reticulocyte count	30%	10%	5%
Platelet count	18%	4%	21%
Increase in marrow blasts	15%	5%	0%

patients experienced improvement in the granulocyte count, 6% in the reticulocyte count, and 2% in the platelet count. Five percent showed progression to acute leukemia.

Toxicity of GM-CSF and G-CSF is similar, even though G-CSF appears to be tolerated much better. Side effects of these two agents include fatigue, a flu-like syndrome, bone pains, rash, anorexia, headaches, and thrombocytopenia. Serious toxicities like hypotension, pulmonary edema, and cardiac arrythmias are seen less often, usually with higher doses.

At present, the dose of 1–3 µg/kg/day for both GM-CSF and G-CSF is considered to be effective and safe. The effect of these agents disappears about 4 weeks after the drug is stopped.

Thus, in summary, the effects of GM-CSF and G-CSF are primarily limited to stimulation of the granulocytic series. The effect on erythroid and megakaryocytic precursors is minimal and not clinically beneficial. The improvement in the granulocyte count is temporary, but it does reduce the risk of infection during therapy. The toxicity of lower doses appears tolerable, and G-CSF appears to be better tolerated than GM-CSF. There is no strong evidence that these agents promote leukemic transformation in myelodysplastic syndromes. Hence, one can justify the use of these agents in patients with granulocytopenia for short periods of time. Long-term use, because of their injectable formulation, cost, and toxicity, is not practical (Table 9.6).

Interleukin-3 (IL-3):   IL-3, also known as *granulocyte-erythroid-macrophage-megakaryocytic colony-stimulating factor (GEMM-CSF),* is a cytokine with broadly stimulatory effect on the common progenitor cells for granulocytic, macrophage, erythroid, and megakaryocytic lines. As a single agent, IL-3 (dose range, 30–1,000 µ/m^2) has been shown to raise granulocyte counts in about 55%, reticulocyte counts in 5%, and platelet counts in 21% of the patients with MDSs. The data, however, remain preliminary, as only a small number of patients with MDS have been treated with IL-3 so far. Side effects of IL-3 are similar to those of other colony-stimulating factors but tend to be milder. A small number of patients may develop thrombocytopenia while on IL-3. There are no reports of leukemic transformation with IL-3 therapy in MDSs (Table 9.6).

IL-6 and IL-11 have the ability to stimulate thrombopoiesis and may have potential—as single agents or in combination—in the management of patients with MDSs. Preliminary data on these agents should soon be available. Stem cell factor also stimulates hematopoiesis in vitro and in primates. Patients with MDSs have also been reported to have lower levels of plasma stem cell factor compared to normal subjects. Therefore, stem cell factor may have utility in the treatment of myelodysplasia. There are no data on the use of stem cell factor in MDSs.

Combinations of Colony-Stimulating Factors: The major purpose of using combinations of colony-stimulating factors is to broaden the scope of hematopoietic stimulation, as many patients are bi- or pancytopenic, and single agents usually provide a lineage-restricted advantage. In addition, in vitro and primate data suggest that the use of two colony-stimulating factors may have a synergistic effect on hematopoiesis. Such synergy was demonstrated between erythropoietin and G-CSF by Greenberg and colleagues (1991) and between IL-3 and GM-CSF by Donohue et al. (1988). Interestingly, the sequential use of IL-3 and GM-CSF gives better results than simultaneous administration of these agents, presumably because they both share the same receptors.

The clinical experience with combinations of colony-stimulating factors is still small and is not very encouraging. Trials using erythropoietin and G-CSF are in progress. In cancer patients, the combination of IL-3 and GM-CSF produced a neutrophilic response that was superior to that seen with single agents, but the effect on the red cells and platelets was not better. Sequential use of these two agents in MDS has confirmed these observations. The toxicity of this combination, however, was substantial, with one-third of the patients developing bone pains and serious cardiac and infectious complications.

The overall outlook for the use of colony-stimulating factors in the management of MDSs remains limited. This may be largely due to the fact that the ineffective hematopoiesis in these patients has only limited potential for expansion and differentiation. Many of the colony-stimulating factors have a lineage-restricted stimulatory effect that may not be clinically beneficial in a given patient. The injectable formulation of these drugs and their high cost hinder their prolonged use. Therefore, one can envisage the use of colony-stimulating factors only in selected circumstances. It will be reasonable to obtain erythropoietin levels in anemic patients with MDS who require red cell transfusion. If the level is under 100 mU/mL, a trial of erythropoietin is justifiable. Similarly, neutropenic patients may be treated with G-CSF to improve their neutrophil counts if they are febrile. Any further use of CSFs should be restricted to clinical trials.

Biological Response Modifiers: Abnormalities of immune reactivity in MDSs have been documented for many years. These include a decrease in NK cell activity and suboptimal interferon production after a challenge with measles virus–infected HeLa cells. In 1986–87, Elias and associates reported improvement in blood counts in patients with MDS treated with interferon alpha. There were two case reports (Galvani 1987, Block 1988) of patients with MDS achieving a complete clonal remission with alpha interferon. Larger phase II studies have failed to show any remarkable responses to alpha interferon therapy (dose, 3 mU/day subcutaneously), with response rates ranging between 5% and 12%. Alpha interferon is quite toxic in patients with myelodysplasia, partly due to the advanced age of these patients. The side effects seen were a flu-like syndrome, lethargy, anorexia, nausea and vomiting, diarrhea, myelosuppression, and liver dysfunction. A significant number of patients developed septic complications, requiring hospital-ization.

Experience with gamma interferon, interleukin-2, and tumor necrosis factor is minimal, and these agents should be used only in clinical trial settings.

List and colleagues (1990) have reported on their experience with cyclosporin A in MDS. Cyclosporin A is an immunosuppressive agent used in organ transplant patients to prevent rejection and in aplastic anemia. A closer look reveals that the patients with MDSs who responded to cyclosporin had hypoplastic bone marrows. Since there is a significant area of overlap between aplastic anemia and MDSs, it is possible that the responders to cyclosporin therapy may have had an aplastic anemia–like disorder.

In general, biological response modifiers do not appear to be effective agents in the treatment of MDSs, and are quite toxic in this patient population. Their use should be limited to clinical trials.

Chemotherapy

Use of chemotherapeutic agents is primarily limited to CMML, RAEB, and RAEB-IT. In the latter two diseases, the leukemic clone has already established itself in the bone marrow and the cytopenias may be quite severe. The clinical problems observed are similar to those seen in acute leukemia. Thus, a patient may have all the complications present in acute leukemia without meeting its diagnostic criteria. Such patients should be treated with acute leukemia therapy. Similarly, patients with CMML may have severe cytopenias and the associated complica-tions, forcing the physician to initiate aggressive treatment.

Single-agent and combination chemotherapy have been tried in MDSs. The agents used are the same as those employed in the treatment of acute leukemia.

Single-Agent Therapy:

Cytarabine: Low-dose cytarabine was initially reported to be useful in MDSs by Baccarani et al. in 1983. Later that year, Wisch and associates reported on responses obtained by continuous infusion of low-dose cytarabine in MDSs. The most defini-tive study on the use of cytarabine in MDS was a randomized trial of low-dose cytarabine versus supportive care alone carried out by the Eastern Co-operative Oncology Group and the Southwest Oncology Group (Miller et al. 1988). A total of 140 patients were entered in the study. Low-dose cytarabine produced 4% complete responses and improvement in blood counts in 15%, but was also associ-ated with a higher incidence of septic complications. The rate of transformation to acute leukemia and overall survival were similar in both groups. The total published experience with low-dose cytarabine includes 250 patients so far. Seven-teen percent of these patients achieved a complete remission, and blood counts improved in another 19%. The median survival was not improved with low-dose cytarabine. Initially, it was believed that low-dose cytarabine acts as a differentia-tion-inducing agent. However, it is now clear that even at low doses, cytarabine functions primarily as a myelotoxic agent.

High-dose cytarabine ($2–3$ g/m^2 every 12 hr for 6 days) was not found to be more effective in a small series of patients reported by Preisler et al. (1986). Only 2 out of 15 patients achieved a complete remission. Toxicity of the therapy was severe and proved fatal in more than 40% of the patients.

Table 9.7   Chemotherapy in MDSs: Response Rates and Survival

Agent	Author	No. of Patients	CR	PR	Median Duration of Survival
		Single-Agent Chemotherapy			
Low-dose cytarabine	Miller	140	8%	15%	8.7 months
High-dose cytarabine	Preisler	15	2%	—	43 days
Low-dose etoposide	Ogata	11	10%	30%	12 months
Homoharringtonine	Feldman	11	20%	10%	—
		Combination Chemotherapy			
Daunomycin + cytarabine	Armitage	20	20%		1 month
Daunomycin + cytarabine	Tricot	15	53%		8 months
Rubidazone + cytarabine	Fenaux	20	50%		6 months
Daunomycin + cytarabine + thioguanine	Aul	16	56%		5 months

Abbreviations: CR = complete response; PR = partial response.

Therefore, cytarabine, in either low or high doses, does not appear to be a useful agent in MDSs.

Other Single Agents: Low-dose azacytidine has already been discussed as a differentiating agent. It is not clear if this agent, like cytarabine, also acts primarily through its myelotoxic effects. Low-dose etoposide, hydroxyurea, oral idarubicin, and homoharringtonine have all been tried in MDS. The data are either anecdotal or preliminary, and the results do not appear to be promising. Further studies will be necessary to determine their role in the management of MDS.

Response and survival rates for single-agent therapy are presented in Table 9.7.

Combination Chemotherapy: The main subgroups treated with combination chemotherapy are RAEB, RAEB-IT, and CMML. Reported series frequently have had small number of patients, and the data from reports with more than 10 patients are summarized in Table 9.7. The combinations utilized were daunomycin plus cytarabine; daunomycin plus high-dose cytarabine; rubidazone plus cytarabine; and daunomycin, cytarabine, and thioguanine. The complete response rates varied between 15% and 56%, but the duration of responses was short, ranging between 1 and 8 months. The treatment-related mortality was disturbingly high, at 13–30% in different series. The overall survival actually appears to be shorter in the treated patients in some studies.

The response rates observed in MDSs are lower than those seen in de novo acute leukemias. The reasons for this difference are unclear. However, data suggest that, at least in some patients, the multiple drug resistence gene (*MDR1*) may be expressed early. By using the *MDR1* gene probe, Holmes et al. (1989) showed that marrow cells from 7 out of 19 patients expressed this gene at diagnosis. Another study (List et al. 1991) showed the presence of p-glycoprotein in 22% of the cases with MDS. Interestingly, the expression of p-glycoprotein, the *MDR1* gene product, was associated with CD34 positivity in these cases. The significance of this association is not known.

Overall, it appears that combination chemotherapy is very toxic and produces only brief complete remissions in MDS. The reasons for this severe toxicity are not entirely clear, but may be related to the advanced age of these patients and the long neutropenic periods induced by the chemotherapy. The use of combination chemotherapy should be restricted to selected patients who have no other options and who are otherwise healthy.

Treatment of Acute Leukemia Evolving from an MDS

AMLs which result from transformation of a myelodysplastic syndrome are, as a rule, less responsive to standard chemotherapy. A review of eight different reports involving 195 patients shows complete response rates of 22% to 62%, with median survival of 5–8 months. Therapeutic regimens used were daunomycin with standard or high-dose cytarabine in most series. The therapy-related death rate was very high, varying between 21% and an amazing 64%. Prolonged neutropenia and the older age of these patients make the therapy particularly hazardous. Interestingly, some patients relapse into their previous myelodysplastic state with chemotherapy.

Bone Marrow Transplantation in MDSs

In patients with a poor prognosis, bone marrow transplantation appears to offer the best chance of a cure at this time. Unfortunately, this option is not available to a majority of these patients, either from lack of appropriate donors or because of the advanced age of the patients. Despite these limitations, a substantial body of literature has been published in this area, with encouraging results.

There are four major reports in the literature on 20, 78, 86, and 93 patients about the use of allogeneic bone marrow transplantation in MDSs (Table 9.8). The upper age limit was 60 years. All FAB subgroups were treated. Preparative regimens for the transplantation were the same as those used for acute leukemias. From 35% to 45% of the patients appear to have obtained durable complete remissions, with follow-up periods that range from 108+ days to 3714+ days. Multivariate analysis of data from some of these studies shows that younger age and shorter disease duration prior to the transplantation were associated with prolonged disease-free survival.

The toxicity of the transplantation is significant, with 22–45% of patients suffering fatal complications from the bone marrow transplantation itself. Younger patients (below 40 years) experienced less toxicity and had better disease-free survival.

Thus, within its limitations, allogeneic bone marrow transplantation may be one of the better treatment modalities for MDSs. It certainly is an attractive option for younger patients who are otherwise in good health and have an appropriately matched donor.

Recently, autologous bone marrow transplantation has been attempted by Laporte et al. (1993) in patients with MDSs after purging the marrow with mafosfamide. Two of the seven patients treated remain in remission at 10 and 28 months after the transplant, demonstrating the feasibility of this approach. Others have demonstrated that polyclonal hematopoiesis is established in patients with MDSs

Table 9.8   Bone Marrow Transplantation in MDSs: Results of Major Trials

Author	No. of Patients	FAB Subtypes	Preparative Regimen	Disease-Free Survival	Follow-up
O'Donnell	20	CMML 2 RAEB 4 RAEBIT 8 Others 5 AML 1	Cyt ± A/TBI	35%	108+ to 3,359+ days
DeWitte	78	RA 9 CMML 1 RAEB 16 RAEBIT 20 sAML 32	Variable	45%	2 years
Sutton	86	RA 20 RAEB 26 RAEBIT 18 sAML 17 Others 5	Cy-TBI Bu-Cy	38%	—
Anderson	93	AA 11 RA 29 RAEB 31 RAEBIT 14 Myelofib 4 CMML 2 Others 2	Cy ± TBI Bu-Cy	41%	4 years

Abbreviations: FAB = French American British; Cy = cyclophosphamide; TBI = total body irradiation; Bu = busulfan; RAEB = refractory anemia with excess blasts; RAEB-IT = RAEB in transformation; CMML = chronic myelomonocytic leukemia; AML = acute myelogenous leukemia; sAML = secondary AML; RA = refractory anemia; AA = aplastic anemia; Myelofib = Myelofibrosis.

after successful chemotherapy, making the possibility of autologous stem cell transplantation real. In vitro studies by Glinsmann-Gibson et al. (1994) have shown that the c-kit ligand, (stem cell factor) both alone and in combination with other colony-stimulating factors, restores multipotent progenitors in MDSs. Therefore, there may be a future role for this agent in autologous stem cell or bone marrow transplant for MDSs.

APPROACH TO THE PATIENT WITH MDS

The above discussion on the treatment of MDS suffers from a major flaw: There is no one good treatment for MDS. The options discussed have either a low response rate or prohibitive toxicity or both. The variability in the clinical course of various FAB subgroups makes treatment planning even more difficult. How is one, then, to approach a patient with a new diagnosis of MDS? We would suggest a systematic approach based on the knowledge of natural history, prognostic factors, laboratory data, and the reported outcomes of available therapies. In younger patients, allogeneic bone marrow transplantation should be considered

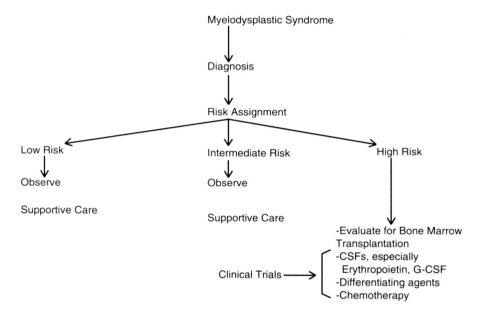

Myelodysplastic Syndrome

Diagnosis

Risk Assignment

Low Risk

Observe

Supportive Care

Intermediate Risk

Observe

Supportive Care

Clinical Trials ⟶

High Risk

-Evaluate for Bone Marrow
Transplantation
-CSFs, especially
  Erythropoietin, G-CSF
-Differentiating agents
-Chemotherapy

Risk Assignment (Hirst WJR, Mufti GJ. Br J Haematol 84: 191–196, 1993)

Low Risk: Monocytopenia (Hg < 10 gm/dl, or absolute neutrophil count of < 2,500/mm^3, or platelet count of < 100,000/mm^3), marrow blast count of < 5%, no ALIP (Abnormal Localization of Immature Precursors), normal marrow cytogenetics or 5q-

Intermediate Risk: Bicytopenia, bone marrow blast count 5–10%, presence of ALIP, simple cytogenetic abnormality or Trisomy 8

High Risk: Tricytopenia, bone marrow blast count > 10%, complex cytogenetic abnormalities, or monosomy 7

Figure 9.2   Approach to a Patient with Myeodysplastic Syndrome

strongly because it is the only potentially curative therapy available at this time. In others, the approach should be conservative, and whenever possible, patients should be treated in clinical trials (Fig. 9.2).

SUMMARY

The clinical features of patients with MDS are not unique and result primarily from the cytopenias. Analysis of data from large series of patients reveals that the bone marrow blast cell count is the most important prognostic factor for survival. In addition, the severity of cytopenias and cytogenetic abnormalities help to determine the prognosis. By using the clinical features and prognostic variables, it is possible to predict the behavior of the disease in broad terms, which, in turn, may help tailor treatment in a given patient. Supportive care remains the mainstay of treatment in MDS. Choice of a definitive therapy can be difficult because there are many options, none of which offer major potential benefit. In younger, otherwise healthy patients, allogeneic bone marrow transplantation should be considered strongly, as this therapy offers the only hope of a cure at this time. The hope, however, must be tempered by knowledge of the toxicity of the procedure and its cost. The timing of the marrow transplantation, especially in slowly evolving cases, may become debatable.

Other patients should be evaluated for treatment with differentiating agents and colony-stimulating factors. The differentiating agents appear to benefit a small number of patients and are relatively nontoxic. Among the colony-stimulating factors, erythropoietin and G-CSF may be useful in selected cases. Erythropoietin should be used in patients with low endogenous levels, and G-CSF should be used for short periods of time to boost the neutrophil count. There is little evidence to recommend the use of steroids, vitamins, or androgens. Use of chemotherapeutic agents should be selective and restricted to high-risk patients with RAEB, RAEB-IT, or CMML. Chemotherapy should be undertaken with the clear understanding that the potential for achieving a complete response is moderate and that the response is usually brief. The toxicity of chemotherapy, on the other hand, is substantial.

BIBLIOGRAPHY

Articles

Anderson JE, Appelbaum FR, Fisher LD, et al: Allogeneic bone marrow transplantation for 93 patients with myelodysplastic syndrome. *Blood* 82:677–681, 1993.

Andreef M, Stone R, Michaeli J, et al: Hexamethylene bisacetamide in myelodysplastic syndrome and acute myeloid leukemia. A phase II trial with a differentiation inducing agent. *Blood* 80:2604–2609, 1992.

Antin JH, Smith BR, Holmes W, et al: Phase I/II study of granulocyte-macrophage colony stimulating factor in aplastic anemia and myelodysplastic syndrome. *Blood* 72:705–712, 1988.

Armitage JO, Dick FR, Needleman SW, et al: Effect of chemotherapy on dysmyelopoietic syndrome. *Cancer Treat Rep* 65:601–605, 1981.

Aul C, Gatterman N, Schneider W: Age related incidence and other epidemiological aspects of myelodysplastic syndromes. *Br J Haematol* 82:358–367, 1992.

Aul C, Schneider W: The role of low dose cytarabine and aggressive chemotherapy in advanced myelodysplastic syndromes. *Cancer* 64:1812–1818, 1989.

Baccarani M, Zaccaria A, Bandini G, et al: Low dose cytarabine for treatment of myelodysplastic syndromes and subacute myeloid leukemias. *Cancer Res* 7:539–545, 1983.

Bagby GC, Gabourel JD: Glucocorticoid therapy in preleukemic syndrome. *Ann Intern Med* 92:55–58, 1980.

Barton JC, Conrad ME, Parmley RT: Acute lymphoblastic leukemia in idiopathic refractory sideroblastic anemia. *Am J Hematol* 9:109–115, 1980.

Block WL, Lowenberg, Sizoo W. Disappearance of trisomy 8 after alpha interferon in a patient with myelodysplastic syndrome. *N Eng J Med* 318:787–788, 1987.

Bowen D, Yancik S, Bennett L, et al: Serum stem cell factor in patients with myelodysplastic syndromes. *Br J Haematol* 85:63–66, 1993.

Cazzola M, Barosi G, Gobbi PG, et al: Natural history of idiopathic refractory sideroblastic anemia. *Blood* 71:305–312, 1988.

Cines DB, Cassileth PA, Kiss JE: Danazol therapy in myelodysplasia. *Ann Intern Med* 103:58–60, 1985.

Clarke RE, Jacobs A, Lush CJ, et al: Effect of 13 cis-retinoic acid on survival of patients with myelodysplastic syndrome. *Lancet* 1:763–765, 1987.

Coiffier B, Adeleine P, Viola JJ, et al: Dysmyelopoietic syndrome. A search for prognostic factors in 193 patients. *Cancer* 52:83–90, 1983.

De Planque MM, Kluin Nelemens HC, van Krieken HJM, et al: Evolution of acquired aplastic anemia to myelodysplasia and subsequent leukemia in adults. *Br J Haematol* 70:55–62, 1988.

DeWitte T, Zwaan F, Hermans J, et al: Allogeneic bone marrow transplantation for secondary acute leukemia and myelodysplastic syndrome: A survey by the Leukemia Working Party of the European Bone Marrow Transplantation Group (EBMTG). *Br J Haematol* 74:151–155, 1990.

Donohue RE, Seehra J, Metzger M, et al: Human interleukin-3 and granulocyte-macrophage colony stimulating factor act synergistically in stimulating hematopoiesis in primates. *Science* 241:1820–1823, 1988.

Economopoulos T, Stathakis N, Karakassis D, et al: Prognostic factors in myelodysplastic syndromes (abstract). *Blut* 56:29A, 1988.

Elias L, Hoffman R, Boswell J: Trial of recombinant alpha interferon in myelodysplastic syndrome. *Leukemia* 1:105–110, 1987.

Eng C, Farraye FA, Shulman LN, et al: The association between myelodysplastic syndrome and Crohn's disease. *Ann Intern Med* 117:661–662, 1992.

Feldman E, Ahmed T, Mittelman A, et al: Phase II trial of homoharringtonine in patients with myelodysplastic syndrome and myelodysplastic syndrome evolving to acute nonlymphoblastic leukemia (abstract). *Proc Am Soc Clin Oncol* 10:228a, 1991.

Fenaux P, Beucart R, Lai JL, et al: Prognostic factors in adult chronic myelomonocytic leukemia. An analysis of 107 cases. *J Clin Oncol* 6:1417–1424, 1988.

Fenaux P, Estienne MH, Lepelley P, et al: Refractory anemia according to the FAB classification. Report on 69 cases. *Eur J Haematol* 40:318–325, 1988.

Fenaux P, Lai JL, Jouet JP, et al: Aggressive chemotherapy in adult primary myelodysplastic syndromes. *Blut* 57:297–302, 1988.

Foucar K, Langdon RM, Armitage JO, et al: Myelodysplastic syndromes: A clinical and pathologic analysis of 109 cases. *Cancer* 56:553–561, 1985.

Galvani DW, Cawley JC, Nethersell, et al. Alpha interferon in myelodysplasia. *Br J Haematol* 66:145–146, 1988.

Ganser A, Seipelt G, Lindemann A, et al: Effect of recombinant human IL-3 in patients with myelodysplastic syndromes. *Blood* 76:455–461, 1990.

Ganser A, Volkens B, Greher J, et al: Recombinant human granulocyte-macrophage colony stimulating factor in patients with myelodysplastic syndromes. A phase I/II trial. *Blood* 73:31–37, 1989.

Ganser A, Lindemann A, Ottmann OG, et al: Sequential in vivo treatment with 2 recombinant human growth factors (IL-3 and GM-CSF) as a new therapeutic modality to stimulate hematopoiesis. Results of a phase I study. *Blood* 79:2583–2589, 1992.

Garcia S, Sanz MA, Amigo V, et al: Prognostic factors in chronic myelodysplastic syndromes. A multivariate analysis of 107 cases. *Am J Hematol* 27:163–168, 1988.

Geissler K, Balent P, Mayer P, et al: Recombinant human IL-3 expands pool of circulating hematopoietic progenitor cells in primates. Synergism with human granulocyte-macrophage colony stimulating factor. *Blood* 75:2305–2311, 1990.

Glinsmann-Gibson B, Spier C, Baier M, et al: Mast cell growth factor (c-kit ligand) restores growth of multipotent progenitors in myelodysplastic syndrome. *Leukemia* 8:827–832, 1994.

Gold EJ, Mertelsman RH, Itri LM, et al: Phase I trial of cis retinoic acid in myelodysplastic syndromes. *Cancer Treat Rep* 67:981–986, 1983.

Greenberg BR, Durie BG, Barnett TC, et al: Phase I/II study of cis-retinoic acid in myelodysplastic syndromes. *Cancer Treat Rep* 69:1369–1374, 1985.

Greenberg PL, Negrin RS, Ginzton N, et al: Granulocyte colony stimulating factor synergizes with erythropoietin for enhancing erythroid colony formation in myelodysplastic syndrome (abstract). *Blood* 78:38a, 1991.

Hellstrom E, Robert KH, Gahrton G, et al: Therapeutic effect of low dose cytarabine, alpha interferon, 1a dihydroxyvitamin D_3 and retinoic acid in acute leukemia and myelodysplastic syndromes. *Eur J Haematol* 40:449–459, 1988.

Herrmann F, Lindemann A, Klein H, et al: Effect of recombinant granulocyte macrophage colony stimulating factor in patients with myelodysplastic syndromes with excess blasts. *Leukemia* 3:335–338, 1989.

Hirst WJR, Mufti GJ: Clinical annotation: Management of myelodysplastic syndromes. *Br J Haematol* 84:191–196, 1993.

Holmes J, Jacobs A, Carter G, et al: Multidrug resistence in haematopoietic cell lines, myelodysplastic syndromes and acute myeloid leukemia. *Br J Haematol* 72:40–44, 1989.

Ito T, Ohashi H, Kagami Y, et al: Recovery of polyclonal hematopoiesis in patients with myelodysplastic syndromes following successful chemotherapy. *Leukemia* 8:839–843, 1994.

Jacobs R, Combleet MA, Vardiman JW, et al: Prognostic implications of morphology and karyotype in primary myelodysplastic syndrome. *Blood* 67:1765–1772, 1986.

Kizaki M, Koeffler HP: Differentiation inducing agents in the treatment of myelodysplastic syndromes. *Semin Oncol* 19:95–105, 1992.

Koeffler HP, Heitjen D, Mertelsman R, et al: Randomized study of 13 cis-retinoic acid versus placebo in myelodysplastic disorders. *Blood* 71:703–708, 1988.

Kurzrock R, Estey E, Talpaz M, et al: All trans-retinoic acid: Tolerance and biologic effects in myelodysplastic syndromes. *J Clin Oncol* 11:1484–1495, 1993.

Kurzrock R, Talpaz M, Estrov Z, et al: Phase I study of interleukin-3 in patients with bone marrow failure. *J Clin Oncol* 9:1241–1247, 1991.

Laporte JP, Isnard F, Lesage S, et al: Autologous bone marrow transplantation with marrow purged by mafosfamide in seven patients with myelodysplastic syndromes in transformation (AML-MDS): A pilot study. *Leukemia* 7:2030–2033, 1993.

Leoni F, Ciolli S, Longo G, et al: 13-cis-retinoic acid treatment in patients with myelodysplastic syndrome. *Acta Haematol* 80:8–12, 1988.

Lessin LS: Multicenter trial demonstrates potential benefit of rHuEPO in MDS. *Peer to Peer* 1:14–19, 1991.

Wang S: Can myelodysplasia evolve into aplastic anemia? *Br J Haematol* 81:450–451, 1992.

Wisch JS, Griffin JD, Kufe DW: Response of preleukemic syndromes to continuous infusion of low dose cytarabine. *N Engl J Med* 309:1599–1602, 1983.

Yoshida Y, Hirashima K, Asano S, et al: A phase II trial of recombinant human granulocyte colony stimulating factor in myelodysplastic syndromes. *Br J Haematol* 78:378–384, 1991.

Yunis J, Lobell M, Arneson MA, et al: Refined chromosome study helps define prognostic subgroups in most patients with myelodysplastic syndromes and acute myelogenous leukemia. *Br J Haematol* 68:184–189, 1988.

Review Articles

Annotation: Is aplastic anemia a preleukemic disorder? *Br J Haematol* 77:447–452, 1991.

Beris P: Primary clonal myelodysplastic syndromes. *Semin Hematol* 26:216–233, 1989.

Cheson BD: The myelodysplastic syndromes. Current approaches to therapy. *Ann Intern Med* 112:932–941, 1990.

Cheson BD: Chemotherapy and bone marrow transplantation for myelodysplastic syndromes. *Semin Oncol* 19:85–94, 1992.

Ganser A, Hoelzer D: Clinical course of myelodysplastic syndromes. *Hematol Oncol Clin North Am* 6:607–632, 1992.

Greenberg PL: Treatment of myelodysplastic syndromes with hematopoietic growth factors. *Semin Oncol* 19:106–114, 1992.

Heim S: Cytogenetic findings in primary and secondary myelodysplastic syndromes. *Leuk Res* 16:43–46, 1992.

Kampmeier P, Anastasi J, Vardiman JW: Issues in the pathology of myelodysplastic syndromes. *Hematol Oncol Clin North Am* 6:501–522, 1992.

Kantarjian HM, Keating MJ: Therapy related leukemia and myelodysplastic syndrome. *Semin Oncol* 14:435–443, 1987.

Koeffler HP, Golde DW: Human preleukemia. *Ann Intern Med* 93:347–353, 1980.

Kouides PA, Bennett JM: Morphology and classification of myelodysplastic syndromes. *Hematol Oncol Clin North Am* 6:485–500, 1992.

List AF, Garewal HS, Sandberg AA: The myelodysplastic syndromes: Biology and implications for treatment. *J Clin Oncol* 8:1424–1441, 1990.

Levine EG, Bloomfield CD: Leukemias and myelodysplastic syndromes secondary to drug, radiation, and environmental exposure. *Semin Oncol* 19:47–84, 1992.

Mecucci C, Van der Berghe H: Cytogenetics. *Hematol Oncol Clin North Am* 6:523–542, 1992.

Noel P, Tefferi A, Pierre RV, et al: Karyotypic analysis in primary myelodysplastic syndromes. *Blood Rev* 7:10–18, 1993.

CASE 1

PATIENT: A 63-year-old woman of Hispanic descent.

CHIEF COMPLAINT: Easy fatigue on exertion.

MEDICAL HISTORY: The patient presented to her physician 3 years ago with easy fatigability. Physical examination was normal. A CBC done at that time showed that she was anemic, with a hemoglobin level of 8.2 g/dL. WBC and platelet counts were normal. Bone marrow examination showed the presence of ringed sideroblasts. Her hemoglobin count gradually fell, and packed red cell transfusions became necessary once a month over the previous year. She was seen by us for a second opinion. Family, personal, and past histories were unremarkable.

PHYSICAL EXAMINATION: A flow-type ejection systolic murmur. Liver span 8 cm by percussion. No splenomegaly.

LABORATORY RESULTS

A. *Screening Procedure*
   WBC 4.4×10^9/L with 72% neutrophils, 23% lymphocytes, 3% monocytes, 1% eosinophils, and 1% basophils. Hg 7.4 g/dL, MCV 98.7 fL, MCH 32.5 pg, MCHC 33.9 g/dL, RDW 24.9%. Platelet count 149×10^9/L. Examination of the blood smear showed some dimorphism and hypochromia of the red cells. Siderocytes were also seen (Case 1.1). A chemistry profile was remarkable for mild elevations of AST (48 IU/L), ALT (82 IU/L), GGT (46 IU/L), and LDH (244 IU/L). Serum folate and vitamin B_{12} levels were normal.

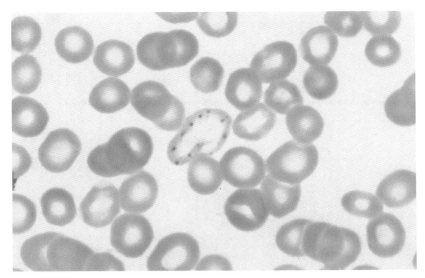

Case 1.1 A dimorphic population of red cells and a siderocyte (center) PB (×1,000).

QUESTIONS

1. What further studies are necessary to establish a diagnosis?
2. Can her clinical course be predicted from the routine studies?
3. Discuss the differential diagnosis of her bone marrow findings.
4. How should she be treated? Will additional studies help design a better treatment plan?

LABORATORY RESULTS

B. *Confirmatory Studies*
    A bone marrow aspirate and biopsy were obtained. Bone marrow was 100% cellular. Erythroid precursors were megaloblastoid and showed nuclear dyskinesis (Case 1.2). Iron stores were increased, and 30% of the erythroid progenitors were ringed sideroblasts (Case 1.3). The blast count was 2%. The bone marrow biopsy showed the presence of a true (MPEX-positive) ALIP, as seen in Case 1.4. Chromosomal analysis of the marrow showed a normal female karyotype. The serum erythropoietin level was 108 IU/mL (normal, less than 15).

DIAGNOSIS: RARS.

CLINICAL COURSE AND THERAPY: At the time of her diagnosis, the patient was treated with oral pyridoxine, 100 mg/day, and folic acid, 1 mg/day, with no improvement in her hemoglobin level. She was subsequently treated with recombinant erythropoietin, 150 U/kg subcutaneously, three times a week for 2 months, with no beneficial effect. Oral cis-retinoic acid, 10 mg/m²/day, was also ineffective. She was subsequently entered into a study protocol which utilized sequential therapy with IL-3 and GM-CSF. With this therapy, her granulocyte and

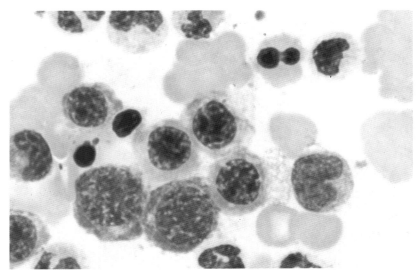

Case 1.2   Megaloblastoid erythroid precursors and nuclear dyskinesis BM (×1,000).

platelet counts improved, but her hemoglobin level remained unchanged. To date, she has received about 80 packed red cell units.

The patient also remains unusually susceptible to infections, developing frequent respiratory infections. During a visit to Mexico she developed pneumonia, which progressed to gram-positive septicemia and renal failure. The patient is currently on chronic hemodialysis. Repeated treatment with erythropoietin has not changed her red cell transfusion requirements.

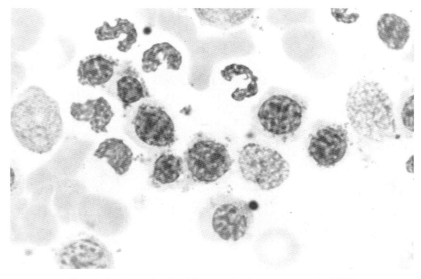

Case 1.3   Ringed sideroblasts in the bone marrow (×1,000).

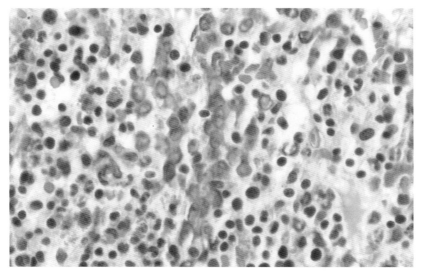

Case 1.4 Bone marrow biopsy showing true (MPEX-positive) ALIP (×400).

DISCUSSION: RARS is one of the more "benign" subgroups of MDS. A majority of the patients are in their 70s at the time of diagnosis. Almost all patients with this diagnosis are anemic, and about one-third also have neutropenia or thrombocytopenia. About 70% of the patients become dependent on red cell transfusions.

The blood smear in RARS may show evidence of dyserythropoiesis and dysgranulopoiesis. At times, erythrocytic dimorphism may be seen (both hypochromic and normally hemoglobinized erythrocytes). The diagnosis of RARS is established by the presence of ringed sideroblasts in the bone marrow, which must account for 15% or more of the nucleated erythroid precursors. The ringed sideroblasts should have five or more ferritin granules that encircle two-thirds of the nucleus (see Chapter 2). Sideroblasts with fewer than five granules are not considered pathological. The blast count in the bone marrow is less than 5%.

The pathogenesis of primary acquired RARS remains obscure. The pathological erythroblasts contain coarse iron granules in the mitochondria. The cause of this intramitochondrial deposition of iron is unclear. Though abnormalities of heme synthesis, and occasionally of cellular respiratory mechanisms, have been demonstrated in some cases, such defects are not seen consistently. Some authors have suggested that primary RARS may be a disorder of mitochondrial DNA.

The main differential diagnosis of RARS is the secondary forms of sideroblastic anemias. These may result from alcohol abuse, lead poisoning or as toxicity of antitubercular drugs like isoniazid or cycloserine. Sideroblastic anemia has also been seen with the use of nitrogen mustard, melphalan, and azathioprine. The presence of ringed sideroblasts has been described in myeloproliferative disorders, lymphomas, autoimmune disorders like systemic lupus erythematousus, and myxedema. Rarely, sideroblastic anemia occurs as a hereditary condition. Both the X-linked and autosomal recessive forms have been described.

The natural history of RARS is indolent. The reported median survival varies between 16 and 76 months, with a mean of about 44 months. Patients who become transfusion dependent do less well, with a survival of 1 to 3 years. Iron overload from repeated red cell transfusions becomes an important cause of morbidity and mortality in these patients. The overall risk of leukemic transformation in RARS is reported to be between 0% and 19%. This risk appears to be higher in patients who have neutropenia and/or thrombocytopenia.

The analysis of prognostic factors in this patient is interesting. As mentioned in Chapter 9, these factors can be given scores to assign patients to low-, intermediate-, or high-risk groups. This patient has a single cytopenia, normal bone marrow cytogenetics, and a blast count of 2% in the bone marrow. These factors put her in the low-risk category. However, she has true (MPEX-positive) ALIP in the marrow. Thus, her overall risk in terms of leukemic transformation and survival worsens to the intermediate group.

The therapy received by this patient seems reasonable. Pyridoxine and folic acid, as expected, did not help her. The use of recombinant erythropoietin can be questioned, as her endogenous erythropoietin levels were more than 100 IU/mL. As discussed in Chapter 9, erythropoietin therapy is less likely to help patients with an adequate erythropoietin response to their anemia. Nevertheless, a short trial to obviate the need for red cell transfusions appears justified. IL-3 and GM-CSF improved her granulocyte and platelet counts. However, these improvements were not clinically meaningful, and the treatment was stopped.

Thus, this patient will remain dependent on supportive therapy. In time, when she has received about 100 U of packed red cells, iron overload will become an issue of clinical importance. She may have to be considered for iron chelation therapy. If she progresses to acute leukemia, her outlook will be quite poor. Chemotherapy may induce a short-term remission, but the risk of fatal toxicity during treatment is high. Because of her age and other medical problems, she is not a candidate for allogeneic bone marrow transplantation.

SUMMARY

Morphology	**Peripheral blood film: Siderocytes in peripheral blood. Bone marrow aspirate: Erythroid precursors with megaloblastoid changes and nuclear dyskinesis. Iron stain ++++. Thirty percent of the erythroid precursors are ringed sideroblasts.**
	Bone marrow biopsy: shows true (MPEX-positive) ALIP.
Cytogenetics	**46XX.**
Chemistry profile	**Serum folate and vitamin B$_{12}$ levels: normal.**
	Serum erythropoietin: 108 IU/mL.
Diagnosis	**RARS**

ANSWERS

1. Clinical evaluation and initial laboratory studies showed a macrocytic anemia which is not due to folate or vitamin B$_{12}$ deficiency. A bone marrow test with a cytogenetic study would be the obvious next step. Cytogenetic studies show an abnormality in about 50% of cases and are helpful in assessing the future course of the disease.

2. Routine studies have only limited power for predicting the outcome in MDS.

However, when combined with bone marrow findings and cytogenetic analysis, they provide a reasonable assessment of the future course of the disease. A schema (see Fig. 9.2) can be constructed, and the patient can be assigned to the low-, intermediate-, or high-risk group.

3. The bone marrow in this case shows two main features: ringed sideroblasts and ALIP. The ringed sideroblasts can be seen in a variety of conditions, such as alcohol abuse, lead poisoning, use of antitubercular drugs, chemotherapeutic agents, lymphomas, thyroid disorders, and so on. In most of these situations, the sideroblasts (and sideroblastic anemia) will resolve if the offending agent is withdrawn or the underlying disorder is treated. In contrast, RARS is an idiopathic, acquired condition which is a preleukemic state. As mentioned earlier, more than 15% of the erythroid precursors must be ringed sideroblasts to make the dignosis of RARS. Therefore, in an anemic patient with ringed sideroblasts in the bone marrow, a thorough search for an underlying pathology should be made, and a diagnosis of RARS should be made by exclusion.

ALIP is present in the bone marrow of virtually all patients with blast counts of 5% or higher. Therefore, in patients with a blast count of less than 5%, presence of a true (MPEX-positive) ALIP is an important finding. Multiple studies have shown that the presence of ALIP is a poor prognostic sign; these patients have a shorter survival and a higher rate of leukemic transformation.

4. Supportive therapy remains the mainstay of treatment for patients with RARS. However, therapies to alleviate the symptomatic cytopenias should be instituted. Since this patient is dependent on red cell transfusions, obtaining an erythropoietin level is important. If it is less than 100 IU/mL, erythropoietin therapy is frequently helpful and may save the patient from complications of iron overload. Use of differentiation-inducing agents and CSFs may be justified. The former are beneficial in a small number of patients, but are relatively nontoxic. The latter may be useful in treating granulocytopenia for short durations.

BIBLIOGRAPHY

Articles

Bennett JM, Catovsky D, Daniel MT, et al: Proposals for classification of myelodysplastic syndromes. *Br J Haematol* 51:189–199, 1982.
Bottomley SS: Sideroblastic anemia. *Clin Haematol* 11:389–394, 1981.
Cartwright GE, Deiss A: Sideroblasts, siderocytes, and sideroblastic anemia. *N Engl J Med* 292:185–188, 1975.
Cazzola M, Barosi G, Gobbi PG, et al: Natural history of idiopathic refractory sideroblastic syndrome. *Blood* 71:305–312, 1988.
Cheng DS, Kushner JP, Wintrobe MM: Idiopathic refractory sideroblastic anemia. Incidence and risk factors for leukemic transformation. *Cancer* 44:724–730, 1979.
Frisch B, Bartl R: Bone marrow histology in myelodysplastic syndromes. *Scand J Haematol* 45(Suppl 45):21–37, 1986.
Juneja SK, Imbert M, Sigaux F, et al: Prevalence and distribution of ringed sideroblasts in primary myelodysplastic syndromes. *J Clin Pathol* 36:1129–1137, 1983.

May A, de Souza P, Barnes K, et al: Erythroblast iron metabolism in sideroblastic marrows. *Br J Haematol* 52:611–621, 1982.

Shafer AI, Cheron RG, Dluhy R, et al: Clinical consequences of acquired transfusional iron overload in adults. *N Engl J Med* 304:319–324, 1981.

Tricot G, De Wolf-Peeters C, Vlietinck R, et al: Bone marrow histology in myelodysplastic syndromes. Prognostic value of ALIP. *Br J Haematol* 58:217–225, 1984.

Wickramsinghe SN, Hughes M: Capacity of ringed sideroblasts to synthesize nucleic acids and proteins in patients with primary acquired sideroblastic anaemia. *Br J Haematol* 38:345–352, 1978.

Review Articles

Cheson BD: The myelodysplastic syndromes: Current approaches to therapy. *Ann Intern Med* 112:932–941, 1990.

Goasguen JE, Bennett JM: Classification and morphologic features of myelodysplastic syndromes. *Semin Oncol* 19:4–13, 1992.

Gattermann N, Aul C, Schneider W: Is acquired sideroblastic anemia a disorder of mitochondrial DNA? *Leukemia* 7:2069–2076, 1993.

Hirst WJR, Mufti GJ: Clinical annotation: Management of myelodysplastic syndromes. *Br J Haematol* 84:191–196, 1993.

Levine EG, Bloomfield CD: Leukemias and myelodysplastic syndromes secondary to drug, radiation, and environmental exposure. *Semin Oncol* 19:47–84, 1992.

List AF, Garewal HS, Sandberg AA: The myelodysplastic syndromes: Biology and implications for management. *J Clin Oncol* 8:1424–1441, 1990.

CASE 2

PATIENT: A 44-year-old Caucasian woman.

CHIEF COMPLAINT: Easy fatigue upon usual exertion (running 5 miles a day) for 1 month.

MEDICAL HISTORY: Except for recent fatigue, the patient had no complaints. Her past and personal histories were unremarkable. One of her nieces died of acute lymphoblastic leukemia. She did not drink alcohol, smoke, or have any exposure to benzene-containing chemicals. There was no exposure to radiation. The patient is an aerobic exercise instructor.

PHYSICAL EXAMINATION: The patient appeared pale. An ejection-type systolic murmur could be heard over the precordium; otherwise, the physical examination was normal.

LABORATORY RESULTS

A. *Screening Procedure*
    WBC 2.2×10^9/L, with 69% neutrophils, 30% lymphocytes, and 1% monocytes; Hg 5.2 g/dL, MCV 95.6 fL, MCH 32.4 pg, MCHC 33.8 g/dL, platelets 141×10^9/L. Examination of the blood smear showed the presence of macro-ovalocytes and teardrop cells (Case 2.1). A chemistry profile showed low cholestrol (121 mg/dL) and elevated LDH of 258 IU/L but was otherwise normal. A sucrose hemolysis test to rule out PNH was normal. The serum folate level was 16.1 ng/mL and the vitamin B_{12} level was 645 pg/mL. The referring physician had done a bone marrow test, which showed dysplastic changes of the erythroid series and approximately 10% blast cells. The marrow cytogenetics had reportedly shown the 5q− abnormality.

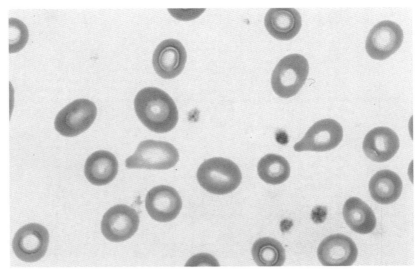

Case 2.1   Peripheral blood smear showing macro-ovalocytes and teardrop cells (×1,000).

QUESTIONS

1. What is the diagnosis by the FAB classification?
2. Does the patient have the so-called 5q− syndrome? How does that affect her future outlook?
3. What is the significance of her chromosomal abnormality? Is this abnormality restricted to MDSs?

LABORATORY RESULTS:

B. *Confirmatory Studies*

A bone marrow examination was performed. The aspirate showed megaloblastoid changes of the erythroid series. An occasional giant band was also seen. The megakaryocytic abnormalities were remarkable, showing vacuolated and mononuclear forms (Cases 2.2 and 2.3). The blast cell count was 8%. Stainable iron was + + + +, but ringed sideroblasts were not seen. Bone marrow biopsy showed a fat:cell ratio of 50:50 and the presence of true (MPEX-positive) (ALIP). Bone marrow cytogenetics showed an interstitial deletion of chromosome 5 (del 5q, q13.q33)

DIAGNOSIS: RAEB (with 5q−)

CLINICAL COURSE: The patient has required packed red cell transfusions every 3–4 weeks since her diagnosis was made. She has been treated with oral pyridoxine, recombinant erythropoietin in a dose of 150–300 U/kg three times a week for 2 months, oral cis-retinoic acid, and IL-3 plus GM-CSF, without any benefit. She has no human leukocyte antigen (HLA)-matched sibling and refuses to be considered for a unrelated allogeneic bone marrow transplantation. She is currently being treated with IL-2.

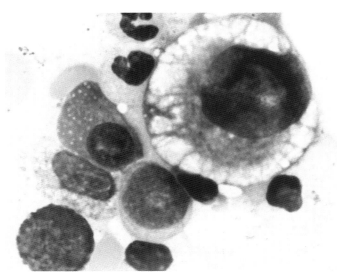

Case 2.2   Bone marrow aspirate showing an immature, vacuolated megakaryocyte (×1,000).

After she had received about 100 U of red cells, a serum ferritin level was obtained and found to be markedly elevated at 2498 ng/mL. A chemistry profile showed abnormal liver function tests. Deferoxamine therapy was begun, but the patient was unable to tolerate it.

DISCUSSION: This patient has RAEB with 5q−. She does not have the 5q− syndrome as it was initially reported in the literature. The 5q− syndrome was first described in 1974 by Van den Berghe in an Italian immigrant in Belgium.

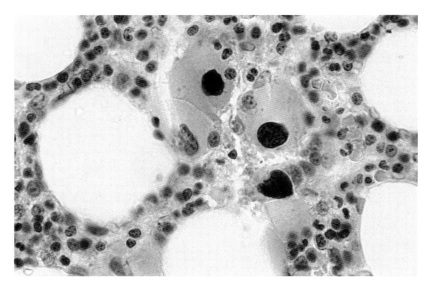

Case 2.3   Mononuclear megakaryocytes in the bone marrow biopsy specimen (×1,000).

Subsequent papers suggested that a refractory anemia with this cytogenetic abnormality may be a separate clinicopathological entity. The patients tend to be predominantly female and have macrocytic anemia, a normal or low WBC count, and thrombocytosis. The bone marrow typically shows decreased erythroid precursors and megakaryocytes with nonlobated nuclei. The characteristic interstitial deletion of the long arm of chromosome 5 is seen on cytogenetic analysis. The clinical course of the 5q− syndrome (RA in the FAB classification) tends to be relatively benign. The median survival of these patients in the early studies was reported to be about 25 months. In a report of six patients by Mahmood et al. (1979), none showed any hematological changes or leukemic transformation after a 5-year follow-up. One of the larger studies of patients with MDS and 5q− chromosomal abnormality was recently published by Mathew et al. (1993) from the Mayo Clinic and included 43 consecutive patients. Seventy-two percent of the patients had RA, 7% RARS, 16% RAEB, and 5% RAEB-IT. Sixteen percent transformed into acute leukemia, which was uniformly fatal. The projected median survival for the whole group was 63 months. Therapy was generally unsuccessful.

Since the original description of the 5q− syndrome, two variants of this RA have been described: type A and type B. RA with del 5 is now termed *5q− syndrome, type A*. *Type B* refers to patients with this syndrome who have an additional chromosomal abnormality. Only a minority of the patients with type B 5q− syndrome have macrocytic anemia and an elevated platelet count. Another group of patients have a RAEB with 5q−. These patients have a median survival of only 5 months.

To complicate matters further, the 5q− abnormality has also been described in a number of other conditions. These include de novo acute nonlymphoblastic leukemia, myeloproliferative disorders, solid tumors, non-Hodgkin's lymphoma, and acute lymphoblastic leukemia.

Thus, it is unclear if 5q− syndrome is indeed a separate clinical entity. Patients who have an RA and the characteristic cytogenetic abnormality of 5q−(q13.q31) may have an indolent clinical course and little risk of leukemic transformation. Patients with RAEB and 5q− tend to do worse, their clinical course paralleling that seen in other patients with RAEB.

In a study of 80 patients with a deletion of 5q, Le Beau et al. (1986) reported that the breakpoints and the extent of deletion varied among patients. However, these investigators found that band 5q31 was deleted in all patients and termed it the *critical region* for this deletion. A number of genes have been mapped to the critical region (Chapter 7). These include a gene encoding for CD14 (a myeloid antigen), the *EGR1* gene (it encodes for a DNA binding zinc finger protein), the PDGFR gene, the beta-2-adrenergic receptor protein gene, the endothelial cell growth factor gene, and genes for IL-3, GM-CSF, IL-4, and IL-5 (Chapters 7 and 8). As can be seen, these genes encode for proteins that have a major impact on hematopoiesis. It is not clear how the deletion of the critical region causes the disease process. It is possible that deletion of 5q31 leads to a loss of the wild-type allele or causes a decrease in the gene product. These issues, however, need to be resolved by further investigation.

A report by Willman et al. in 1993 suggested that deletion of the *IRF*-1 gene, which maps to chromosome 5q31.1, may be the critical deletion in the pathogenesis of myelodysplasia and leukemia. A subsequent report by Boultwood et al. (1993), however, has shown that in some patients with myelodysplasia, the *IRF*-1 gene is retained. This study included 14 patients (8 had RA, 3 RAEB, 1 RAEB-IT, and 2 AML) with 5q−. By FISH, using an IRF 1 cosmid probe, two patients with RA were found to have retained both copies of this gene. More recently, Le Beau et al. have reported that the smallest commonly deleted region of chromosome 5 in malignant myeloid diseases is about 2.8 megabases in size and contains the *EGR1* gene. These investigators suggest that the *EGR1* gene may be a tumor-suppressor gene.

SUMMARY

Morphology	Peripheral blood film: macro-ovalocytes, tear drop cells. Bone marrow aspirate: megaloblastoid erythropoiesis, occasional giant band, blast count 8%. Iron stain ++++, no ringed sideroblasts Bone marrow biopsy: Fat:cell ratio 50:50. True (MPEX-positive) ALIP seen.
Cytogenetics	Del 5 (q13–q33).
Sucrose hemolysis	Negative.
Chemistry profile	LDH: elevated. Cholesterol: decreased. Serum folate and vitamin B_{12}: normal.
Diagnosis	RAEB with 5q−

ANSWERS

1. RAEB.
2. The patient does not have the so-called 5q− syndrome. Since this chromosomal abnormality has been seen in many hematological malignancies and solid cancers, it will be best to restrict the diagnosis of 5q− syndrome to patients who have this cytogenetic abnormality and the clinical features described in the original publications, i.e., macrocytic anemia, normal or low WBC count, thrombocytosis, and nonlobated megakaryocytes in the bone marrow. Could she have had this syndrome to begin with and evolved to RAEB subsequently? As mentioned in the Discussion section, Mahmood et al. (1979) did not find any such progression in their patients after a 5-year follow-up. Thus, it is unlikely, though possible, that the patient evolved into RAEB from RA with the 5q− syndrome.

   Her future outlook is similar to that of patients with RAEB. As mentioned in Chapter 9, one of the most important ominous prognostic factors in MDSs is a marrow blast percentage of 5% or higher. The patients prognosis is poor because her marrow blast percentage is 8%. Patients who have RAEB with 5q− syndrome have a median survival of only about 5 months.
3. The chromosomal abnormality seen in this patient is obviously very significant. As mentioned in the Discussion, all patients with 5q− have a deletion of the 5q31 band, which contains a large number of genes encoding for proteins directly affecting hematopoiesis.

   The presence of 5q− is not restricted to RA. It has also been seen in patients with RAEB, acute leukemia, myeloproliferative disorders, lymphomas, and solid tumors.

BIBLIOGRAPHY

Articles

Boultwood J, Fidler C, Lewis S, et al: Allelic loss of *IRF*-1 in myelodysplasia and acute myeloid leukemia. Retention of *IRF*-1 on the 5q− chromosome in some patients with 5q− syndrome. *Blood* 82:2611–2616, 1993.

Le Beau M, Espinoza R, Neuman WL, et al: Cytogenetic and molecular delineation of the smallest commonly deleted region of chromosome 5 in malignant myeloid diseases. *Proc Natl Acad Sci USA* 90:5484–5488, 1993.

Le Beau M, Lemons RS, Espinosa R, et al: Interleukin-4 and interleukin-5 map to human chromosome 5 in a region encoding growth factors and receptors, and are deleted in myeloid leukemias with a del(5q). *Blood* 73:647–650, 1989.

Le Beau M, Pettenati MJ, Lemons RS, et al: Assignment of GM-CSF, CSF-1, and FMs genes to human chromosome 5 provides evidence for linkage of a family of genes regulating hematopoiesis and their involvement in the deletion of 5q in myeloid disorders. *Cold Spring Harbor Symp Quant Biol* 51:899, 1986.

Mahmood T, Robinson WA, Riddell B, et al: Macrocytic anemia, thrombocytosis, and nonlobulated megakaryocytes. The 5q− syndrome. A distinct entity. *Am J Med* 66:946–950, 1979.

Mathew P, TefferiA, Dewald GW, et al: The 5q− syndrome: A single institution study of 43 consecutive patients. *Blood* 81:1040–1045, 1993.

Nagarajan L, Zavadil J, Claxton D, et al: Consistent loss of D5S89 locus mapping telomeric to the interleukin gene cluster and centromeric to *EGR*-1 in patients with 5q− chromosome. *Blood* 83:199–208, 1994.

Nand S, Sosman J, Godwin J, et al: A phase I/II study of sequential interleukin-3 and granulocyte-macrophage colony stimulating factor in myelodysplastic syndromes. *Blood* 83:357–360, 1994.

Swohn B, Weinfeld A, Riddell B, et al: The 5q− deletion: Clinical and cytogenetic observations in ten patients and review of the literature. *Blood* 58:986–993, 1981.

Van der Berghe H, Cassiman JJ, David G, et al: Distinct haematological disorder with deletion of long arm of No. 5 chromosome. *Nature* 251:437–438, 1974.

Willman C, Sever C, Pallavicini MG, et al: Deletion of *IRF*-1, mapping to chromosome 5q31.1, in human leukemia and preleukemic myelodysplasia. *Science* 259:968–971, 1993.

Review Articles

Beris P: Primary clonal myelodysplastic syndromes. *Semin Hematol* 26:216–233, 1989.

Cheson BD: The myelodysplastic syndromes. Current approaches to therapy. *Ann Intern Med* 112:932–941, 1990.

Greenberg PL: Treatment of myelodysplastic syndromes with hematopoietic growth factors. *Semin Oncol* 19:106–118, 1992.

Kampmeier P, Anastasi J, Vardiman JW: Issues in the pathology of the myelodysplastic syndromes. *Hematol Oncol Clin North Am* 6:501–522, 1992.

Van den Berghe H: The 5q− syndrome. *Scand J Haematol* 36(Suppl 45):78–81, 1986.

PATIENT: A 69-year-old Caucasian woman.

CHIEF COMPLAINT: Easy fatigue for 3 months. Weight loss of 40 lb. in the previous 6 months.

MEDICAL HISTORY: The patient was seen by another physician 2 years earlier for an abnormal CBC, which was discovered accidentally. She was diagnosed as having an early phase of myelofibrosis with myeloid metaplasia (MMM) and was started on oral hydroxyurea. She remained asymptomatic until 3 months ago, when she developed easy fatigability. Her father had died from sarcoma and her mother from colon carcinoma. She had smoked for 100 pack-years, but had not been exposed to unusual chemicals.

PHYSICAL EXAMINATION: Total liver span by percussion was 12 cm, and a spleen tip was felt on deep inspiration. The physical examination was otherwise unremarkable.

LABORATORY RESULTS

A. *Screening Procedure*
WBC 8.8×10^9/L, HGB 10.8 g/dL, MCV 100.5 fL, MCH 33.7 pg, MCHC 33.5 g/dL, platelets 6.6×10^9/L. Differential count showed 13% blasts, 57% neutrophils, 20% lymphocytes, 4% reactive lymphocytes, and 6% monocytes. Examination of the blood smear showed the presence of both type I and II blasts (Case 3.1). Rare teardrop cells were seen. The chemistry profile was significant for a lactose dehydrogenase (LDH) level of 314 IU/L. A bone marrow examination done by the referring physician showed an increased number of promyelocytes in the marrow.

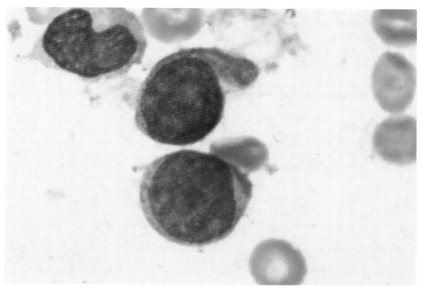

Case 3.1 Type I and type II blasts (type I blast, lower) in the peripheral blood smear (×1,000).

QUESTIONS

1. What is your diagnosis from the data presented?
2. How often does MMM evolve into myelodysplasia? Is the natural history of this "secondary MDS" different from that of de novo MDS?
3. Is the possibility of acute promyelocytic leukemia (APL) real in this case? How often does APL present initially as MDS? Or, stated another way, how often does MDS evolve into APL?
4. What further studies will help resolve the issues raised in question 3?
5. What would be the appropriate management in this case?

LABORATORY RESULTS

B. *Confirmatory studies*

A bone marrow examination was performed. The aspirate was easily obtained and showed hypercellularity. The blast count was 21%. Numerous promyelocytes were also seen, raising the possibility of APL (Cases 3.2, 3.3). However, no Auer rods or faggot cells were observed. Bone marrow biopsy showed a fat:cell ratio of 20:80. Reticulum stain was moderately positive. The bone marrow was submitted for a cytogenetic analysis. This showed a normal female karyotype. Special stains (MPEX+, SBB+, A-EST+, B-EST−, CAE+, C-EST some CAE with fluoride resistance, some A-EST with fluoride sensitivity) showed that the blasts belonged to the myeloid (M4) lineage. In our experience, B-EST, although very specific, is not as sensitive as A-EST. Flow

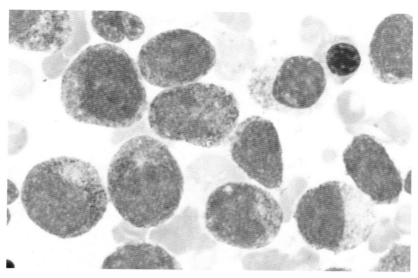

Case 3.2   Many promyelocytes are seen in the bone marrow smear, raising the possibility of APL. However, no Auer rods or faggot cells are seen. Note some cells with few or no granules which represent blasts. (×1,000).

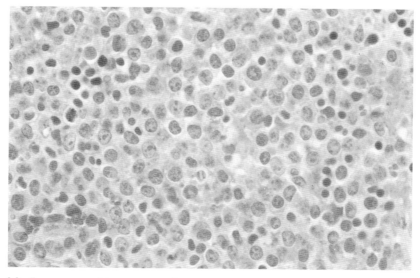

Case 3.3   Bone marrow biopsy smear shows numerous immature cells which probably represent promyelocytes and blasts. Exact differentiation between blasts and promyelocytes can be difficult at times by hematoxylin-eosin biopsy preparation (×400).

cytometry showed that the marrow cells were predominantly CD11c/LEUM5 (94%) and CD34/HPCA2 (87%) positive.

DIAGNOSIS: RAEB-IT

CLINICAL COURSE AND THERAPY: Hydroxyurea therapy was continued and cis-retinoic acid was added. The patient was cautioned about the likelihood of her disease progression to AML. Three months later, she developed a rapidly progressive pneumonia and died of respiratory failure in 7 days.

DISCUSSION: This patient is interesting from many aspects. She was initially diagnosed as having MMM, which apparently was in its early phase at that time. After 2 years, her disease evolved into RAEB-IT. She died soon afterward; very likely from progression of her disease.

Myelofibrosis results from excessive release of platelet-derived growth factor (PDGF) from the abnormal platelets and megakaryocytes of patients with MMM. There is some evidence that this may result from activation of the oncogene *c-sis* on chromosome 22. About 5% of patients with MMM transform into acute leukemia. The reported interval to leukemic transformation ranges from 14 to 48 months. Though the authors have personally taken care of patients with MMM who developed RAEB and RAEB-IT, there are no reports about the incidence of these complications in MMM. Because of dry bone marrow aspirates and the tendency of the blasts to cluster, precise morphological diagnosis becomes quite difficult in such cases.

This patient was given hydroxyurea. The leukemogenic potential of this drug is not known. In the Polycythemia Vera Study Group (Kaplan et al. 1986), use of hydroxyurea was associated with a 5.9% risk of leukemic transformation in patients with polycythemia vera. Compared to historical controls, this risk was not statistically significant. Thus, it is not clear if hydroxyurea played any role in the evolution of this patient's illness.

The diagnosis of RAEB-IT in this case was based on the percentage of blasts in the peripheral blood and/or bone marrow. The peripheral blood blast percentage varied from 13% to 21%, with the higher percentages reported during infections (a blast percentage of 30% or more in the peripheral blood is diagnostic of acute leukemia). An intriguing feature of this case was the presence of promyelocytes on the blood smear and their increased percentage in the marrow, raising the possibility of APL. This possibility was later discounted by the special stains and by the absence of 15,17 translocation. The presentation of APL as an MDS has been reported in the literature in rare cases, and the authors have also diagnosed such a case. This patient presented with pancytopenia and was diagnosed as having RA. However, the marrow cytogenetics showed the characteristic 15,17 translocation. The patient evolved into a typical APL in 7 months.

The flow cytometric data in this patient provided important prognostic information. There are many reports about the surface markers of the bone marrow cells in MDSs, as well as their association with the incidence of leukemic transformation and survival in these patients. The following antigens have been studied: Ia (HLA-DR), CD11b (Mo 1), CD13 (My7), CD14 (Mo2, My4), CD15, CD33 (My9), and CD34. High HLA-DR and low CD11b expression was found to be associated with early conversion to acute leukemia. CD34 was found to be the only independent predictor of poor survival. The presence of CD34+ cells in peripheral blood in patients with MDSs has also been reported to be a adverse prognostic feature.

The patient's thrombocytopenia and blast count put her in a high-risk category of MDS. The therapeutic options were limited. There is obviously no role for hematopoietic growth factors. The addition of cis-retinoic acid was of no benefit. Antileukemic chemotherapy would have been the next obvious step, but the patient died from a septic complication before such therapy could be instituted. Because of her age, she was not a candidate for bone marrow transplantation.

SUMMARY

Morphology	**Peripheral blood film: Showed the presence of both type I and type II blasts. Occasional teardrop cells.**
	Bone marrow aspirate: Numerous promyelocytes. Blast count 21%. The blasts were MPEX+, SBB+, A-EST+, some A-EST with fluoride sensitivity, B-EST−, CAE+, some CAE with fluoride resistance.
	Bone marrow biopsy: Fat:cell ratio 20:80. Reticulum stain moderately positive.
Bone marrow flow cytometry	**CD11c/LEUM5 94%, CD34/HPCA2 87%.**
Bone marrow cytogenetics	**46XX.**
Chemistry profile	**LDH elevated.**
Diagnosis	**RAEB-IT.**

ANSWERS

1. RAEB-IT.

2. The true incidence of transformation of MMM into MDS is not known. As mentioned earlier, about 5% of the patients with MMM will transform into acute leukemia. Many of these patients will pass through a preleukemic phase, as the process of transformation is often slow. The natural history of this secondary MDS has not been well defined.

3. The morphology was very suggestive of the possibility of APL in this case. This, however, was easily ruled out by special stains and the cytogenetics. Evolution of MDS to APL is rare, as is evolution to acute lymphoblastic, bilineal, and biphenotypic leukemia.

4. Patients with APL frequently have a bleeding diathesis at presentation because of disseminated intravascular coagulation. Bone marrow and, at times, peripheral blood show the presence of promyelocytes. Auer rods are usually seen. The special stains and, to some extent, flow cytometric characteristics (lack of HLA-DR antigen expression) help distinguish APL from other subtypes. Cytogenetic analysis, with FISH technique to detect the 15,17 translocation, have become very specific and sensitive methods to make a diagnosis of APL. Virtually all patients with APL have the 15,17 translocation. It is very important to make the diagnosis of APL quickly, as it has therapeutic implications. Such patients can achieve complete remission with oral all-trans-

retinoic acid, which is less toxic than chemotherapy and does not require a long hospitalization.

5. A trial of differentiation-inducing agents will be reasonable in this patient. If the disease continues to progress, chemotherapy should be started. The patient is above the age limit for bone marrow transplantation.

BIBLIOGRAPHY

Articles

Ellis JT, Peterson P, Geller SA, et al: Studies of the bone marrow in polycythemia vera and the evolution of myelofibrosis and second hematologic malignancies. *Semin Hematol* 23:144–155, 1986.

Guyotat D, Campos L, Thomas X, et al: Myelodysplastic syndromes: A study of surface markers and in vitro growth patterns. *Am J Hematol* 34:26–31, 1990.

Hasselbalch H: Idiopathic myelofibrosis: A clinical study of 80 patients. *Am J Hematol* 34:291–300, 1990.

Kaplan ME, Mack K, Goldberg JD, et al: Long term management of polycythemia vera with hydroxyurea. A progress report. *Semin Hematol* 23:167–171, 1986.

Lambertenghi-Deliliers G, Orazi A, Luksch R, et al: Myelodysplastic syndrome with increased marrow fibrosis. A distinct clinicopathologic entity. *Br J Haematol* 78:161–166, 1991.

Meng-er H, Yu-chen Y, Shu-rong C, et al: Use of all-trans-retinoic acid in the treatment of acute promyelocytic leukemia. *Blood* 72:567–572, 1988.

Michels SD, Saumur J, Arthur DC, et al: Refractory anemia with excess of blasts in transformation: Hematologic and clinical study of 52 patients. *Cancer* 64:2340–2346, 1989.

Miller JB, Testa JR, Lindgren V, et al: The pattern and clinical significance of karyotype abnormalities in patients with idiopathic and post-polycythemic myelofibrosis. *Cancer* 55:582–591, 1985.

Mittelman M, Karcher DS, Kammerman LA, et al: High HLA la (HLA-DR) and low CD11b expression may predict early conversion to leukemia in myelodysplastic syndromes. *Am J Hematol* 43:165–171, 1993.

Stone RM, Mayer RJ: The unique aspects of acute promyelocytic leukemia. *J Clin Oncol* 8:1913–1921, 1990.

Sullivan SA, Marsden KA, Lowenthal RM, et al: Circulating CD+34 cells: An adverse prognostic factor in the myelodysplastic syndromes. *Am J Hematol* 39:96–101, 1992.

Review Articles

Grignani F, Fagioli M, Alcalay M, et al: Acute promyelocytic leukemia: From genetics to treatment. *Blood* 83:10–25, 1994.

Kampmeier P, Anastasi J, Vardiman JW: Issues in the pathology of myelodysplastic syndromes. *Hematol Oncol Clin North Am* 6:501–522, 1992.

StockW, Larson RA: Managing myelodysplasia. *Contemp Oncol* 1:41–48, 1991.

Ward HP, Block MH: The natural history of agnogenic myeloid metaplasia and a critical evaluation of its relationship with the myeloproliferative syndrome. *Medicine* 50:357–411, 1971.

PATIENT: A 31-year-old Caucasian male.

CHIEF COMPLAINT: Fatigue and easy bruising for 2 years.

MEDICAL HISTORY: The patient was seen by another physician for fatigue and easy bruising 2 years ago. CBC showed pancytopenia. A bone marrow aspirate and biopsy performed at that time showed both hypoplasia and dysplasia of the hematopoietic elements. The patient did not take any medications, and there was no history of exposure to any unusual chemicals or radiation. The family history was unremarkable. He had been treated with prednisone, antithymocyte globulin, and GM-CSF without success. He was now seen for a second opinion for his pancytopenia.

PHYSICAL EXAMINATION: Petechiae were seen around both ankles; otherwise, the physical examination was normal.

LABORATORY RESULTS

A. *Screening procedure*

CBC done 2 years earlier showed WBC count of 1.2×10^9/L with 1% bands, 43% neutrophils, 55% lymphocytes, 1% monocytes, HGB 4.1 g/dL, and platelets 13×10^9/L. Now (the patient was on oral prednisone at this time) the CBC showed WBC 2.7×10^9/L (12% neutrophils, 1% monocytes, and 87 lymphocytes), HGB 11.1 g/dL (after transfusion), MCV 107.6 fL, MCH 37.2 pg, MCHC 34.5 gm/dL, RDW 18.6%, and platelet count 12×10^9/L. Blood smear showed macrocytes. The bone marrow exam from 2 years ago showed complete aplasia in some areas. Other areas were 30–40% cellular, and showed nuclear dyskinesis and megaloblastoid changes.

199

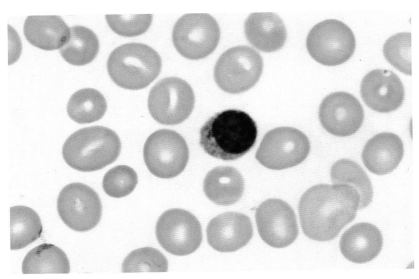

Case 4.1   Macrocytes. Note their size in relation to that of the small lymphocyte. WBC and platelet counts were decreased. PB (×1,000).

QUESTIONS

1. Does this patient have aplastic anemia or MDS? How can these disorders be distinguished from each other?
2. Does aplastic anemia evolve into MDS? How often does it happen and why?
3. What is the natural history of patients with hypoplastic myelodysplasia?
4. If patients have both hypoplasia and dysplasia of the marrow, how should they be treated?

LABORATORY RESULTS

B. *Confirmatory Studies*

Examination of the peripheral blood smear showed the presence of macrocytes, as well as decreased WBCs and platelets (Case 4.1). The bone marrow aspirate and biopsy were repeated, showing nuclear dyskinesis and megaloblastoid changes (Case 4.2) and aplasia (Case 4.3). Some areas of the marrow were more cellular. The overall fat:cell ratio was about 10:90. The blast count was 2%. A cytogenetic study could not be performed, as the marrow specimen did not contain enough cells. Bone marrow cytogenetics done on the first specimen revealed del 16. The sucrose hemolysis test was negative. Serum folate and vitamin B_{12} levels were normal.

DIAGNOSIS: Hypoplastic RA.

CLINICAL COURSE AND THERAPY: The patient was treated with a combination of IL-3 and GM-CSF. No significant improvement in the hemoglobin level or the platelet count was observed. The neutrophil count improved to $5.64 \times 10^9/$L. Because of significant toxicity, the therapy could not be continued. The patient was referred for unrelated bone marrow transplantation, as he had no siblings.

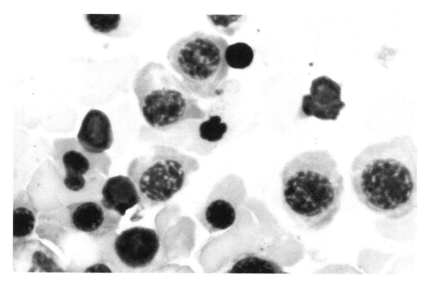

Case 4.2 Bone marrow aspirate showing megaloblastoid erythroid precursors and nuclear dyskinesis (×1,000).

DISCUSSION: This patient has features of both aplastic anemia and MDS. Even in the early 1950s, it was recognized that a small number of patients with aplastic anemia would evolve into MDSs and acute leukemia. Over the next 20 years, it was reported that 1–3% of patients with an initial diagnosis of aplastic anemia would undergo this transformation. It is also well known that patients with PNH, a clonal disorder of the bone marrow stem cells, can present with a hypoplastic

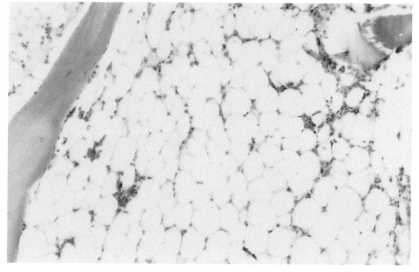

Case 4.3 Bone marrow biopsy specimen showing an area of aplasia (×400).

bone marrow and have a high risk of leukemic transformation. In 1988, Nand and Godwin described a series of patients with features of marrow hypoplasia and dysplasia. The hypoplastic variant constituted about 16% of the total number of patients with MDSs and included patients with RA, RARS, and RAEB. Patients with hypoplastic MDSs tended to have lower WBC and platelet counts, and their red cells showed macrocytic indices. There was no significant difference in the incidence of leukemic transformation or survival. Therapy, whether intended for aplastic anemia or myelodysplasia, was generally unsuccessful.

Over the last few years, it has become increasingly clear that there is a significant overlap between aplastic anemia and MDSs. Van Kamp and associates (1991), by analyzing the RFLPs of the X-linked genes of patients with acquired aplastic anemia, have shown that 13 out of 18 (72%) patients with acquired aplastic anemia had clonal hematopoiesis. Long-term follow-up on patients also seems to support these findings. Tichelli et al. (1992) followed a group of 117 patients with acquired aplastic anemia for 14 years. Eleven patients developed MDSs and 17 developed PNH. The authors determined that the risk of developing a clonal hematopoietic disorder in aplastic anemia at 10 years is 42%. An European Co-operative Group study of 223 patients with aplastic anemia showed that at 7 years after diagnosis, there is a 13% risk of developing PNH and a 15% risk of developing an MDS or acute leukemia. Similar data were reported in a Swiss study of 103 patients (De Planque MM et al., 1989). However, it must be remembered that over the last 15 years, patients with aplastic anemia have been treated with more intensive immunosuppressive therapy than in the past. This has included antithymocyte globulin and cyclosporine in addition to corticosteroids. At this time, it is unclear if immunosuppressive therapy has any role in the development of clonal or malignant hematopoietic disorders in these patients.

There is, thus, strong evidence that in a significant number of patients, aplastic anemia is the initial phase of an ongoing disease process that will subsequently prove to be either a clonal preleukemic disorder or an acute leukemia. Therefore, PNH must be ruled out in all patients who present with aplastic anemia. Whether other studies, like flow cytometric or cytogenetic analysis of the marrow, should be routinely done in aplastic anemia patients at the time of diagnosis is debatable. In the authors' opinion, these studies should be done at the outset. This may help identify a subgroup that is at higher risk of transforming to a clonal or malignant hematological disorder. It may also help clarify the role of immunosuppressive agents in aplastic anemia.

We believe that this patient has hypoplastic MDS. Even though the marrow is severely hypoplastic, morphological evidence of dysplasia is easily seen. The cytogenetic abnormality, though atypical, supports this diagnosis. Finally, the patient did not respond to any form of therapy for aplastic anemia. Though this is no proof, it does not negate the contention that this patient's primary problem is myelodysplasia.

The treatment of this patient has been appropriate. It will be reasonable to try cyclosporine plus prednisone in the future. In addition, erythropoietin levels should be obtained. If they are below 100 IU/mL, erythropoietin therapy may raise his hemoglobin level and obviate the need for red cell transfusions. None of these measures, however, is likely to prolong his survival. As this patient is young, bone marrow transplantation must be considered, as it is the only treatment providing long-term remission. Since he has no siblings, the possibility of an unrelated marrow transplant should be explored.

SUMMARY

Morphology	Peripheral blood film: Macrocytes, leukopenia, thrombocytopenia. Bone marrow aspirate: Hypoplastic marrow with megaloblastoid changes and nuclear dyskinesis of erythroid series. Blast cell count 2%. Iron stain ++++. No ringed sideroblasts. Bone marrow biopsy: Overall fat:cell ratio 90:10.
Cytogenetics	Del 16.
Sucrose hemolysis test	Negative.
Serum vitamin B_{12} and folate levels	Normal.
Diagnosis	Hypoplastic RA.

ANSWERS

1. This patient has an MDS with hypoplastic bone marrow. This diagnosis is based on the presence of macrocytes in the blood, dysplastic changes in the marrow, and abnormal cytogenetics. Aplastic anemia results from an overall decrease in the number of stem cells in the marrow, which may be caused by any of numerous insults, such as radiation, drugs, viral infections, and immune system injury. In many instances, the cause of aplastic anemia cannot be found. The blood picture is that of pancytopenia, and the bone marrow is hypoplastic. The marrow cells, as a rule, do not show megaloblastic or dysplastic changes. The karyotype in aplastic anemia is usually normal; if abnormal, it does not show karyotypic abormalities associated with the MDSs. Nevertheless, some cases may be impossible to categorize precisely.

2. As mentioned in the discussion, the distinction between aplastic anemia and MDS may not be sharp in a significantly large number of patients. Earlier studies indicated that 1–3% of the patients with aplastic anemia may evolve into an MDS or acute leukemia. More recent studies put this risk at 28–42%. Even more startling is the fact that in a small study, 78% of the patients with acquired aplastic anemia were found to have clonal hematopoiesis.

3. Hypoplastic forms of MDS are seen primarily in the RA, RARS, and RAEB subgroups of MDSs. Hypoplastic acute leukemia has also been described. There appears to be no difference in the natural history of hypoplastic variants of the different FAB subgroups compared to those with normo- or hypercellular marrows.

4. Since therapy for aplastic anemia is so successful and that for the MDSs is not, all patients should be initially treated as having aplastic anemia. All patients should be screened for PNH, and erythropoietin levels should be obtained. In the authors' opinion, cytogenetic and flow cytometric analyses should also be performed. If a suitable donor is available, bone marrow transplantation should be considered early. If not, therapy with cyclosporine and prednisone or antithy-

mocyte globulin and prednisone should be tried. Combinations of CSFs can be an equally effective therapy. If these measures fail, other treatment modalities which are usually tried in MDSs should be employed.

BIBLIOGRAPHY

Articles

Coiffier B, Adeleine P, Viala JJ, et al: Dysmyelopoietic syndromes: A search for prognostic factors in 193 patients. *Cancer* 52:83–90, 1983.

De Planque MM, Bacigalupo A, Wursch A, et al: Long term follow up of severe aplastic anaemia patients treated with antithymocyte globulin. *Br J Haematol* 73:121–126, 1989.

De Planque MM, Kluin Nelemens HC, van Krieken HJM, et al: Evolution of acquired aplastic anemia to myelodysplasia and subsequent leukemia in adults. *Br J Haematol* 70:55–62, 1988.

Frisch B, Bartl R: Bone marrow histology in myelodysplastic syndromes. *Scand J Haematol* 36:21–47, 1986.

Gladson CL, Naeim F: Hypocellular bone marrow with increased blasts. *Am J Hematol* 21:15–22, 1986.

Nand S, Godwin JG: Hypoplastic myelodysplastic syndrome. *Cancer* 62:958–964, 1988.

Tichelli A, Gratwohl A, Nissen C, et al: Morphology in patients with severe aplastic anemia treated with anti-thymocyte globulin. *Blood* 80:337–345, 1992.

Tichelli A, Gratwohl A, Wursch A, et al: Late haematological complications in severe aplastic anemia. *Br J Haematol* 69:413–418, 1988.

Tricot G, DeWolf-Peeters C, Hendrickx B, et al: Bone marrow histology in myelodysplastic syndromes. I. Histological findings in myelodysplastic syndromes and comparisons with bone marrow smears. *Br J Haematol* 57:423–430, 1984.

van Kamp H, Landagent JE, Jansen RPM, et al: Clonal hematopoiesis in patients with aplastic anemia. *Blood* 78:3209–3214, 1991.

Yoshida Y, Oguma S, Uchino H, et al: Refractory myelodysplastic anemias with hypocellular bone marrow. *J Clin Pathol* 41:763–777, 1988.

Young NS: The problem of clonality in aplastic anemia: Dr. Dameshek's riddle restated. *Blood* 79:1385–1392, 1992.

Review Articles

Annotation: Is aplastic anemia a preleukemic disorder? *Br J Haematol* 77:447–452, 1991.

Camitta BM, Storb R, Thomas ED: Aplastic anemia. *N Engl J Med* 306:645–652, 1982.

Kampmeier P, Anastasi J, Vardiman JW: Issues in the pathology of myelodysplastic syndromes. *Hematol Oncol Clin North Am* 6:501–522, 1992.

Kouides PA, Bennett JM: Morphology and classification of myelodysplastic syndromes. *Hematol Oncol Clin North Am* 6:485–500, 1992.

CASE **5**

PATIENT: A 37-year-old Caucasian male.

CHIEF COMPLAINT: Weakness and easy bruising for 4 weeks.

MEDICAL HISTORY: The patient sought medical attention for a 4-week history of easy fatigue and easy bruisability. His past and family histories were insignificant. He worked in a tile factory and had no known exposure to unusual chemicals or radiation. He drank six beers a week and had smoked one pack of cigarettes a day for 20 years.

PHYSICAL EXAMINATION: The patient was pale and had multiple cutaneous ecchymoses over his arms and legs. The spleen tip was palpable 1 cm under the left costal margin. The rest of the physical examination was unremarkable.

LABORATORY STUDIES:

A. *Screening Procedure*
    WBC count was 6.6×10^9/L, with 12% blasts, 39% neutrophils, 20% monocytes, 2% eosinophils, 2% basophils, and 25% lymphocytes. Hemoglobin was 4.2 g/dL, MCV 99.8 fL, MCH 30.2 pg, MCHC 34.9%, and RDW 13.3%. Platelet count was 17×10^9/L. The peripheral blood blasts showed the presence of Auer rods (Case 5.1).

QUESTIONS

1. What is your diagnosis?
2. Does this patient have AML?

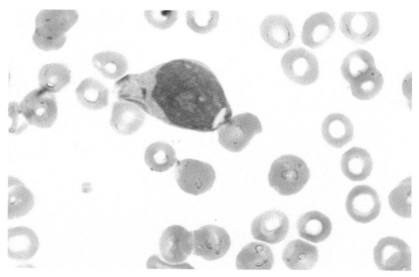

Case 5.1 A type 1 blast with an Auer rod in the peripheral blood (×1,000).

3. What is the significance of splenomegaly in this patient? How often does one find splemomegaly in MDSs?

4. What are the treatment options for this patient? Which one is the best?

CONFIRMATORY STUDIES: Bone marrow examination showed the aspirate to be hypercellular, with 8% blasts. Forty-eight percent of the marrow cells were erythroid precursors and showed megaloblastoid and dysplastic features (Cases 5.2 and 5.3). Iron stain was 2+ positive, but ringed sideroblasts were not seen.

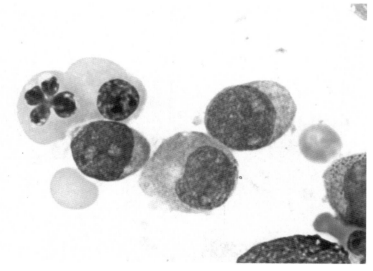

Case 5.2 Bone marrow aspirate showing megaloblastoid changes and nuclear dyskinesis in the erythroid series (×1,000).

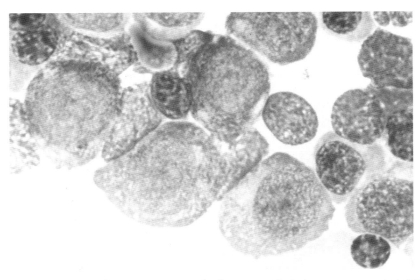

Case 5.3   Megaloblastoid changes in younger red cell precursors in the bone marrow aspirate ($\times$1,000).

The biopsy specimen showed a fat:cell ratio of 1:99. Cytochemical evaluation showed that the blasts were MPEX+, SBB+, and CAE+. Cytogenetic analysis of the bone marrow showed a normal karyotype.

DIAGNOSIS: RAEB-IT.

CLINICAL COURSE AND THERAPY: The patient was admitted to the hospital and was given induction therapy with idarubicin and cytarabine. He achieved a complete remission and was evaluated for an allogeneic bone marrow transplantation. This was carried out a month after completion of his induction therapy. Except for mild graft-versus-host disease, his clinical course has been uncomplicated, and the patient remains in complete remission 9 months after transplantation.

DISCUSSION: This case raises interesting diagnostic and therapeutic questions. The diagnosis is RAEB-IT, based on a blast count of more than 5% in the peripheral blood and the presence of Auer rods in the peripheral blood blasts. As mentioned in Chapter 2, RAEB-IT can be diagnosed by any of the following criteria: peripheral blood blast count of 5% or more (not to exceed 29%), bone marrow blast count of 21–30%, or the presence of unequivocal Auer rods in granulocytic precursors. The last diagnostic criterion is somewhat unusual and was established in 1983, when Weisdorf and associates described five patients who had RAEB but whose blasts showed the presence of Auer rods. To recognize this entity separately, the FAB group included this subgroup in RAEB-IT. The median survival of these patients is 14 months, with a range of 2–27 months. In younger patients (less than 45 years old), this type of RAEB-IT tends to evolve rapidly into acute leukemia.

The history of Auer rods is interesting. These were initially described in 1908 in a patient on Sir William Osler's service and were mistakenly presumed to be present in lymphoblasts. Subsequent observations showed that Auer rods are exclusively seen in AML and at times in blast crisis. The FAB group initially considered the presence of Auer rods as diagnostic of AML, but later rescinded the diagnosis of AML and placed the finding of an unequivocal Auer rod in the RAEB-IT MDS category. The prognostic significance of Auer rods in RAEB-IT is not known. A recent paper by Seymour and Estey (1993) on 208 patients seen between 1973 and 1992 reported that patients diagnosed as having RAEB-IT solely on the basis of the presence of Auer rods had a better survival. The authors in fact suggested that such patients should not be grouped with RAEB-IT patients. Even those patients who had all the other criteria of RAEB-IT and Auer rods had higher response rates to chemotherapy. Thus, the presence of Auer rods appear to bestow a better prognosis in RAEB-IT.

Another intriguing feature of this case is the marked preponderance of erythroid precursors in the marrow. However, the patient does not meet the diagnostic criteria of M6 AML. In M6 AML, the erythropoietic elements account for more than 50% of all nucleated cells in the bone marrow and the myeloblasts constitute 30% of the nonerythroid elements. This patient has 48% erythroid progenitors in the marrow, but his marrow blast count, even after excluding the erythroid elements, is too low to make the diagnosis of acute leukemia. It is possible that, in time, this patient might have progressed to M6 acute myeloid leukemia. Kowal-Vern and associates (1992) have tried to determine the significance of marrow proerythroblasts in patients with FAB M6 AML (previously known as *Di Guglielmo's syndrome*) and Di Guglielmo's disease, in which the bone marrow shows a preponderance of proerythroblasts. The authors found that patients with 30% or more proerythroblasts in the marrow did very poorly, with a median survival of only 2 months. These investigators believe that such patients should not be diagnosed as having MDS and should be included in the FAB M6 AML category.

This patient also had splenomegaly, which is seen in about 17% of all patients with MDSs. It is more common in patients who have marrow fibrosis or a significant degree of ineffective erythropoiesis. Splenomegaly does not appear to have a prognostic implication for patients with MDSs.

The cytogenetic analysis of the marrow cells was normal in this patient. The incidence of karyotypic abnormalities is higher in patients with RAEB and RAEB-IT than in the other subgroups. The types of abnormalities seen are generally similar to those seen in AMLs. They are discussed in detail in Chapter 7. Many studies have shown that deletions involving chromosome 7 and multiple complex abnormalities portend a poor prognosis. Others have shown that cytogenetic abnormalities plus morphological features are of prognostic significance. In some reports, cytogenetic changes were not found to be of independent prognostic value.

The outlook of patients with RAEB-IT is quite poor. The incidence of leukemic transformation has been reported to be 44–67%. This is misleading, as many patients die of complications resulting from the cytopenias without converting into acute leukemia. The median survival reported in various studies ranges from 2.5 to 11 months.

B vitamins, corticosteroids, differentiation-inducing agents, and CSFs are usually not helpful in RAEB-IT. Most clinicians treat this subgroup like acute leukemia. Combination chemotherapy induces complete remissions in 20–50% of patients. Toxicity of the chemotherapy tends to be severe, and remissions are brief. In patients under the age of 60 years, allogeneic bone marrow transplantation remains an attractive choice and may lead to long-term remission in 35–45% of cases.

Recently, it has been shown that it is possible to restore polyclonal hematopoiesis in patients with MDSs after the use of chemotherapy. In vitro marrow culture studies done by Glinsmann-Gibson et al. (1994) reveal that stem cell factor, alone or in conjunction with other CSFs, stimulates the growth of normal pluripotent marrow cells obtained from the marrows of patients with MDSs. A recent study (Laporte et al., 1993) has shown that autologous marrow transplantation, after purging with mafosfamide, is feasible in patients with MDSs. Thus, autologous bone marrow transplants appear to be feasible in patients with MDSs, and autologous stem cell transplants may become possible in the future.

SUMMARY

Morphology	**Peripheral blood film: Twelve percent type 1 blast cells, some containing Auer rods.**
	Bone marrow aspirate: Eight percent type 1 blast cells with erythroid megaloblastoid and dysplastic features.
	Bone marrow biopsy: Marked hypercellularity (99%).
Cytochemistry	**MPEX+, SBB+, CAE+.**
Cytogenetics	**46,XY.**
Diagnosis	**RAEB-IT with increased erythroid elements.**

ANSWERS

1. The diagnosis in this patient is RAEB-IT. This is based on the presence of more than 5% blasts in the peripheral blood and the presence of Auer rods in the circulating blasts.

2. This patient does not have acute leukemia based on the peripheral blood findings. The authors require 30% or more blast cells in the peripheral blood to make a diagnosis of acute leukemia.

3. Splenomegaly is seen in about 17% of patients with MDSs. This may be related to myelofibrosis in the marrow or may result from ineffective erythropoiesis. The patient with dyserythropoiesis may have elevated LDH and bilirubin levels. There is no known clinical significance of splenomegaly in myelodysplasia.

4. The treatment options in this case are limited. Since the patient has life-threatening cytopenias and belongs to an MDS subgroup with a poor outlook, he should be treated aggressively. Because of his younger age, he is a good candidate for marrow transplantation. He was treated with combination chemotherapy initially and obtained a complete remission. Subsequently, an allogeneic bone marrow transplantation was successfully performed. The transplantation gives this man his best chance of achieving long-term remission or cure.

BIBLIOGRAPHY

Articles

Bennett JM, Catovsky D, Daniel MT, et al: Proposals for the classification of acute leukemias. *Br J Haematol* 33:451–458, 1976.
Del Potro E, Martinez R, Krsnik I, et al: Myelofibrosis in primary myelodysplastic syndromes. *Br J Haematol* 73:281–287, 1989.
Foucar K, Langdon RM, Armitage JO, et al: Myelodysplastic syndromes: A clinical and pathologic analysis of 109 cases. *Cancer* 56:533–561, 1985.

Frisch B, Bartl R: Bone marrow histology in myelodysplastic syndromes. *Scand J Haematol* 36(Suppl 45):21–37, 1986.

Glinsmann-Gibson B, Spier C, Baier M, et al: Mast cell growth factor (c-kit ligand) restores growth of multipotent progenitors in myelodysplastic syndrome. *Leukemia* 8:827–832, 1994.

Ito T, Ohashi H, Kagami Y, et al: Recovery of polyclonal hematopoiesis in patients with myelodysplastic syndromes following successful chemotherapy. *Leukemia* 8:839–843, 1994.

Kowal-Vern A, Cotelingam J, Schumacher HR: The prognostic significance of proerythroblasts in acute erythroleukemia. *Am J Clin Pathol* 98:34–40, 1992.

Laporte JP, Isnard F, Lesage S, et al: Autologous bone marrow transplantation with marrow purged by mafosfamide in patients with myelodysplastic syndromes in transformation (AML-MDS): A pilot study. *Leukemia* 7:2030–2033, 1993.

Pagliuca A, Layton DM, Manoharan A, et al: Myelofibrosis in primary myelodysplastic syndromes. A clinicopathologic study of 10 cases. *Br J Haematol* 71:499–504, 1989.

Seymour JF, Estey EH: The prognostic significance of Auer rods in myelodysplasia. *Br J Haematol* 85:67–76, 1993.

Todd WM, Pierre RV: Preleukemia: A long term prospective study of 326 patients. *Scand J Haematol* 45:114–120, 1986.

Weisdorf DJ, Oken MM, Johnson J, et al: Chronic myelodysplastic syndrome: Short survival with or without evolution to acute leukemia. *Br J Haematol* 55:691–700, 1983.

Review Articles

Beris P: Primary clonal myelodysplastic syndromes. *Semin Hematol* 26:216–233, 1989.

Cheson BD: Myelodysplastic syndromes. Current approaches to therapy. *Ann Intern Med* 112:619–632, 1990.

De Witte T, Gratwohl A: Bone marrow transplantation for myelodysplastic syndrome and secondary leukemias. *Br J Haematol* 84:361–364, 1993.

Kampmeier P, Anastasi J, Vardiman JW: Issues in pathology of myelodysplastic syndromes. *Hematol Oncol Clin North Am* 6:501–522, 1992.

Kouides PA, Bennett JM: Morphology and classification of myelodysplastic syndromes. *Hematol Oncol Clin North Am* 6:485–500, 1992.

Loffler H, Schmitz N, Gassman W: Intensive chemotherapy and bone marrow transplantation for myelodysplastic syndromes. *Hematol Oncol Clin North Am* 6:619–632, 1992.

CASE **6**

PATIENT: A 56-year-old Caucasian woman.

CHIEF COMPLAINT: Weakness and easy bruising for 4 months.

MEDICAL HISTORY: The patient has a 36-year history of rheumatoid arthritis, for which she received conventional therapy until 11 years ago, when cyclophosphamide was begun. Her dose varied from 50 to 100 mg/day. After 6 years, cyclophosphamide therapy was stopped because of the concern about delayed toxicity. Four years later, a routine CBC revealed pancytopenia. Bone marrow examination was performed, and the patient was informed that her marrow did not "produce enough cells and showed scarring." Subcutaneous erythropoietin injections were begun but did not help. Over the next 6 months, the blood counts worsened and the patient required platelet and red cell transfusions. She was seen at our institution for a second opinion.

Besides rheumatoid arthritis, the patient has had diabetes mellitus for 35 years and coronary artery disease for 4 years. There was no history of exposure to industrial chemicals or radiation in the past.

PHYSICAL EXAMINATION: Multiple bruises were seen over all four extremities; otherwise, the examination was normal. In particular, there was no lymphadenopathy or hepatosplenomegaly. Remarkably, the joints did not show advanced changes of rheumatoid arthritis.

LABORATORY RESULTS

A. *Screening Procedure*
   CBC showed a WBC count of 4.3×10^9/L, with a differential count of 3% blasts, 2% metamyelocytes, 6% bands, 76% neutrophils, 8% lymphocytes, 2%

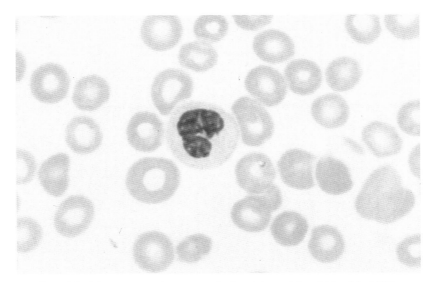

Case 6.1   Macrocytes and an agranular band in peripheral blood (×1,000).

basophils, and 3% eosinophils. HGB was 8.5 g/dL (after transfusion of 2 U of packed red cells), hematocrit 25.2%, MCV 83 fL, MCH 28 pg, MCHC 33.6%, and RDW 15.2%. The platelet count was 36×10^9/L (after an 8-U platelet transfusion). The reticulocyte count was 0.2%. The chemistry profile was unremarkable. Examination of the peripheral blood smear showed the presence of agranular bands and macrocytes (Case 6.1).

QUESTIONS

1. As this patient has a marked left shift of the peripheral blood granulocytes, as well as possible fibrosis of the marrow, could she have a myeloproliferative disorder like CML or myelofibrosis that may be transforming to acute leukemia?
2. How does her long-standing rheumatoid arthritis influence her hematological status?
3. Is her MDS due to her cyclophosphamide therapy? Is the timing right for such a complication to occur?
4. How does secondary or t-MDS differ from de novo MDS?
5. How should this patient be managed now?

LABORATORY RESULTS

B. *Confirmatory Results*

Examination of the bone marrow aspirate revealed 14% blast cells and megaloblastoid erythroid precursors (Case 6.2). Bone marrow biopsy showed a fat cell ratio of 20:80 and extensive fibrosis (Case 6.3). Reticulum stain was +++ positive. Cytogenetic analysis of the bone marrow cells showed del(1) t(1;7)(p11.11) in 100% of the metaphases studied. This abnormality results in loss of chromosomal material from the long arm of chromosome 7 and is frequently associated with therapy-related MDSs or AML.

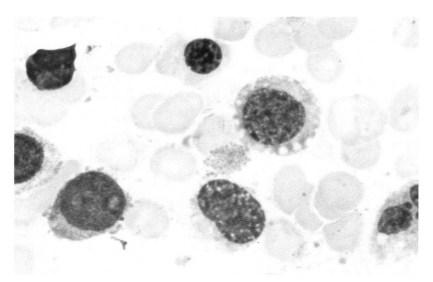

Case 6.2   Bone marrow aspirate showing abnormal and megaloblastoid erythroid precursors and a blast (lower left) (×1,000).

DIAGNOSIS: RAEB (t-MDS).

CLINICAL COURSE: The patient received sequential IL-3 plus GM-CSF therapy on a protocol. Her hemoglobin and platelet count did not improve, and the therapy was discontinued. Chemotherapy was not recommended because of her concomitant medical problems. She was not considered to be a bone marrow

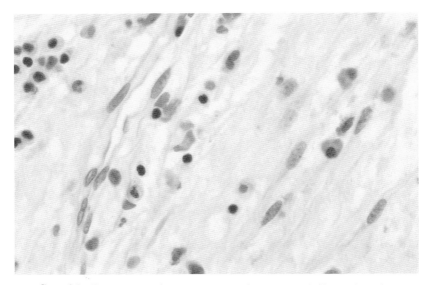

Case 6.3   Bone marrow biopsy specimen showing myelofibrosis (×400).

transplantation candidate for the same reasons. She returned to her family physician for supportive care and was lost to follow-up.

DISCUSSION: This patient almost certainly had a secondary MDS, due to prolonged therapy with cyclophosphamide. The strongest evidence for this diagnosis comes from the cytogenetic studies on her bone marrow. She received an alkylating agent which is known to be associated with secondary myelodysplasia or acute leukemia. The timing of this complication is within the range described. Predictably, her disease did not respond to therapeutic interventions.

Therapy-related MDS or AML (t-MDS or t-AML) can occur after treatment with alkylating agents, procarbazine, nitrosoureas, etoposide, and mitolactol (Chapter 3). It can also occur after radiation and environmental exposure to benzene. The median time from initial treatment to development of t-MDS/AML is 71 months, with a range of 7–331 months. About half of the patients present with an MDS, and about 55% of these progress to acute leukemia. Median survival with secondary MDS is about 45 weeks and, with acute leukemia, 21 weeks. Of those patients who receive chemotherapy, only 29% achieve complete remissions, and these tend to be brief.

The exact pathogenetic mechanisms involved in the evolution of t-MDS or t-AML are not clear. Some investigators have argued that secondary myelodysplasia or leukemia may be part of the natural history of the underlying disease. This argument is supported by the simultaneous and metachronous development of leukemias and other malignancies in patients with untreated breast cancer and chronic lymphocytic leukemia. However, evidence for the leukemogenic potential of irradiation, and of chemotherapeutic agents like alkylators and procarbazine, is very strong and appears to be related to the dose and duration of the offending agent.

Chromosomal abnormalities involving the bone marrow in t-MDS or t-AML predominantly affect chromosomes 5 and 7 and constitute about 43% of all cytogenetic abnormalities seen in these patients. In contrast, only 7% of the karyotypic abnormalities seen in de novo AMLs and 18% of the metachronous leukemias show changes affecting chromosomes 5 and 7. There is also a strong association between the incidence of these abnormalities and the use of certain agents, like melphalan, nitrogen mustard, and nitrosoureas. Some reports have shown that the frequency of chromosome 5 and/or 7 abnormalities may reach 72–83% in patients with Hodgkin's disease, non-Hodgkin's lymphomas, and multiple myeloma treated with alkylating agents and procarbazine.

By combining data from various studies on 216 patients, Bloomfield (1986) reported that 10 abnormal karyotypic patterns can be identified. The karyotypic abnormalities appear to be related to the type of previous malignancy, as well as to previous therapies. When treated for t-MDS or t-AML, patients with 5q− and −5 had the lowest (13%) response rates. Another large study on the cytogenetic characteristics of patients with t-MDS and t-AML was reported by Pedersen-Bjergaard from Denmark (1990). Of the 91 patients studied (62 with MDSs, 29 with AML), 48 had abnormalities involving chromosome 7, 21 involving chromosome 5, 13 involving the short arm of chromosome 17, and 12 involving chromosome 21. In the t-MDS group, the number of chromosomal abnormalities, blast percentage in the marrow, and hemoglobin level were independent prognostic factors.

Though uncommon, balanced translocations involving 11q23 and 21q22 are proving to be very interesting. These are seen in t-MDS or t-AML following therapy with agents that target DNA-topoisomerase II, i.e., doxorubicin, etoposide, and mitoxanterone. These patients have a short interval between treatment and the development of t-MDS or t-AML, and tend to evolve into a M4 or M5a morphology.

This patient's bone marrow showed extensive fibrosis. The issue of myelofibrosis in MDSs is complicated (Chapter 3). In 1981, Sultan and associates described the occurrence of significant myelofibrosis in eight patients with MDSs. Four of them had received previous cytotoxic therapy. Subsequent reports indicate that marked fibrosis occurs in 10–15% of patients, though mild to moderate fibrosis has been described in up to 50%. Myelofibrosis, however, does occur with greater frequency in patients with t-MDS compared to de novo cases. Fibrosis is seen in all five subgroups of MDSs, and the patients tend to have severe cytopenias, hepatomegaly, and splenomegaly. A leukoerythroblastic blood picture is frequently seen. The cause of marrow fibrosis in MDSs remains unclear. Multiple studies have shown that myelofibrosis adversely affects the survival of patients with MDSs. Finally, patients with MDSs with myelofibrosis must be distinguished from those with MMM, later stages of chronic myeloid leukemia, postpolycythemic myelofibrosis, and M7 AML.

This patient had a long history of rheumatoid arthritis, but there was no evidence of Felty's syndrome. Rheumatoid arthritis has no known association with MDSs. A fraction of patients with Felty's syndrome have been reported to have a lymphoproliferative disorder of large granular lymphocytes (LGLs). There is a reported association between patients with LGL lymphoproliferative disorder and other malignancies like AML, myelodysplasia, and plasma cell disorders. The reasons for such associations, uncommon as they are, remain obscure.

SUMMARY

Morphology	**Peripheral blood film: Macrocytosis, agranular granulocytes, 3% blasts.**
	Bone marrow aspirate: Fourteen percent blasts and megaloblastoid precursors.
	Bone marrow biopsy: Marked fibrosis with +++ reticulum stain.
Cytogenetics	**del(1)t(1;7)(p11.11).**
Diagnosis	**RAEB, with myelofibrosis; secondary to therapy with cyclophosphamide (t-MDS)**

ANSWERS

1. The presence of immature granulocytic cells in the blood and the presence of fibrosis in the marrow raise the possibility of a myeloproliferative disorder which may now be transforming into an MDS or acute leukemia. The patient was followed closely by her physicians, and there is no clinical evidence of a myeloproliferative disorder. Absence of splenomegaly also supports this argument. Cytogenetic analysis does not show the presence of a Philadelphia chromosome, but reveals an abnormality of chromosome 7 which is frequently seen in t-MDS or t-AML. Thus, the clinical and laboratory data support the diagnosis of t-MDS.

2. Rheumatoid arthritis is associated with a higher incidence of immune cytopenias (hemolytic anemia, autoimmune neutropenia, and thrombocytopenia). In later stages of the disease, some patients develop Felty's syndrome (splenomegaly, lymphadenopathy, pancytopenia). There is no known association between rheumatoid arthritis and MDSs. Some patients with Felty's syndrome have been known to develop a lymphoproliferative disorder of LGLs. There is a reported association between LGL lymphoproliferative disorder and AML, MDSs, and myeloma.

3. Prolonged cyclosphosphamide therapy is almost certainly responsible for the development of MDS in this patient. Cyclophosphamide is a well-established mutagenic agent, and is known to cause the cytogenetic injury and the clinical disorder that she developed. The reported interval between cytotoxic therapy and development of an MDS is highly variable, ranging from 7 months to 30 years, with a median interval of about 6 years. Therefore, the timing for the development of this complication in this patient is within the described range.

4. Secondary or t-MDSs do not differ significantly from primary MDSs in their clinical presentation. All five FAB subgroups are seen in t-MDSs. Bone marrow fibrosis is seen more frequently in t-MDS. This may lead to a leukoerythroblastic blood picture and a higher incidence of splenomegaly in these patients. A major feature that helps distinguish between t-MDS and primary MDS is the cytogenetic analysis. As mentioned in the discussion (and in Chapters 3 and 7), chromosomes 5 and 7 are frequently involved in t-MDSs, and these abnormalities are considered indirect evidence that exposure to a cytotoxic agent was the likely cause of the MDS. Response rates to therapy and survival of patients with t-MDS are lower than those seen in primary MDS.

5. Given the overall situation of this patient, she should be managed with supportive care only. Her future outlook is bleak.

BIBLIOGRAPHY

Articles

Falkson G, Gelman R, Dreicer R, et al: Myelodysplastic syndrome and acute nonlymphocytic leukemia secondary to mitolactol treatment in patients with breast cancer. *J Clin Oncol* 7:1252–1259, 1989.

Kantarjian HM, Keating MJ, Walters RS, et al: Therapy related leukemia and myelodysplastic syndrome: Clinical, cytogenetic and prognostic features. *J Clin Oncol* 4:1748–1757, 1986.

Michels SD, McKenna RW, Arthur DC, et al: Therapy related acute myeloid leukemia and myelodysplastic syndrome. A clinical and morphologic study of 65 cases. *Blood* 65:1365–1372, 1985.

Ohyashiki K, Ohyashiki JH, Iwabuchi A, et al: Clinical and cytogenetic characteristics of myelodysplastic syndromes developing myelofibrosis. *Cancer* 68:178–183, 1991.

Pedersen-Bjergaard J, Daugaard G, Hansen SW, et al: Increased risk of myelodysplasia and leukemia after etoposide, cisplatin, and bleomycin for germ cell tumors. *Lancet* 338:359–364, 1991.

Pedersen-Bjergaard J, Philip P, Larsen SO, et al: Chromosome aberrations and prognostic factors in therapy-related myelodysplasia and acute nonlymphocytic leukemia. *Blood* 76:1083–1091, 1990.

Pedersen-Bjegaard J, Philip P, Larsen SO, et al: Therapy related myelodysplasia and acute myeloid leukemia. Cytogenetic characteristics of 115 consecutive cases and risk in seven cohorts of patients treated intensively for malignant diseases in the Copenhagen series. *Leukemia* 7:1975–1986, 1993.

Rubin CM, Larson RA, Anastasi J, et al: t(3;21)(q26;q22): A recurring chromosomal abnormality in therapy related myelodysplastic syndrome and acute myeloid leukemia. *Blood* 76:2594–2598, 1990.

Sultan C, Sigaux F, Imbert M, et al: Acute myelodysplasia with myelofibrosis. A report of 8 cases. *Br J Haematol* 49:11–16, 1981.

Third MIC Co-operative Study Group: Morphologic, immunologic and cytogenetic (MIC) working classification for primary myelodysplastic syndromes, therapy related myelodysplasia, and leukemias. *Cancer Genet Cytogenet* 32:1–10, 1988.

Vardiman JW, Le Beau M, Albain K, et al: Myelodysplasia: A comparison of therapy related and primary forms. *Ann Biol Clin (Paris)* 43:369–387, 1985.

Whang-Peng J, Young RC, Lee EC, et al: Cytogenetic studies in patients with secondary leukemia/dysmyelopoietic syndrome after different treatment modalities. *Blood* 71:403–414, 1988.

Review Articles

Bloomfield CD: Chromosome abnormalities in secondary myelodysplastic syndromes. *Scand J Haematol* 36(Suppl 45):82–90, 1986.

Ganser A, Hoelzer D: Clinical course of myelodysplastic syndromes. *Hematol Oncol Clin North Am* 6:543–556, 1992.

Kampmeier P, Anastasi J, Vardiman JW: Issues in the pathology of myelodysplastic syndromes. *Hematol Oncol Clin North Am* 6:501–522, 1992.

Kantarjian HM, Keating MJ: Therapy related leukemia and myelodysplastic syndrome. *Semin Oncol* 14:435–443, 1987.

Schumacher HR, Cotelingam JD: *Chronic Leukemia. Approach to Diagnosis.* New York, Igaku-Shoin, 1993, pp 217–218.

CASE 7

PATIENT: A 64-year-old Caucasian male.

CHIEF COMPLAINT: Easy fatigue and 12-lb weight loss over the previous 3 months.

MEDICAL HISTORY: The patient saw his physician for chest discomfort and was found to have an irregular heartbeat. While awaiting a coronary angiogram due to the possibility of ischemic heart disease, he was found to have an abnormal CBC. He admitted to being tired and losing weight at the time of his evaluation by the hematology service. His past, family, and personal histories were unremarkable. Review of systems revealed that he had had frequent respiratory infections in the previous 2 months. The patient is an attorney and denied having had any exposure to benzene-containing chemicals or any form of radiation.

PHYSICAL EXAMINATION: The physical examination was normal.

LABORATORY RESULTS:

A. *Screening Procedure*
   CBC showed a WBC count of 2.9×10^9/L, with 36% neutrophils, 55% lymphocytes, 5% monocytes, 1% eosinophils, and 3% basophils. Hemoglobin was 11.5 g/dL, HCT 34.2%, MCV 100.4 fL, MCH 30 pg, MCHC 34.7 g/dL, and RDW 15.7%. The platelet count was 101×10^9/L. Examination of the blood smear showed the presence of abnormal immature cells with a convoluted nucleus (Case 7.1). A 300-cell differential on the bone marrow aspirate showed 17% blasts. Agranular bands and nuclear fragmentation in erythroid precursors were seen (Case 7.2). Bone marrow biopsy examination showed areas of hypocellularity, with an overall fat:cell ratio of 90:10 (Case 7.3). Stainable

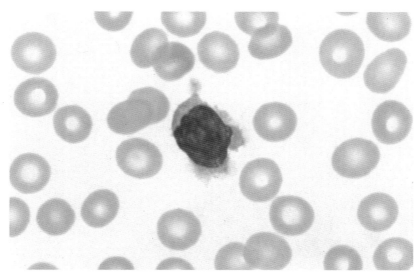

Case 7.1   An immature abnormal cell with a slightly convoluted nucleus PB (×1,000).

iron was increased, and ringed sideroblasts were not seen. Sucrose hemolysis and Ham's tests were negative. Hepatitis B and C screening was negative. The antibody test for parvovirus was negative.

QUESTIONS

1. What further studies are necessary?
2. What is the significance of marrow hypoplasia in this patient? Does it have any bearing on his management?

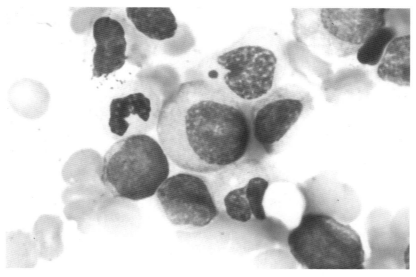

Case 7.2   Bone marrow aspirate showing blasts, agranular bands, and nuclear fragmentation of a red cell precursor (×1,000).

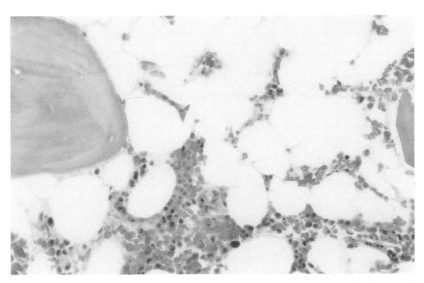

Case 7.3 Bone marrow biopsy showing hypoplasia. Note the small island of cellularity. However, the overall fat:cell ratio was 90:10 (×400).

3. Why does this patient have frequent respiratory infections, despite the fact that his absolute neutrophil count is over $0.5 \times 10^9/L$?

LABORATORY RESULTS

B. *Confirmatory Studies*

Cytochemical studies of the bone marrow showed that the blasts were MPEX+ and SBB+. Other stains could not be performed because of lack of material. Stainable iron was increased, but ringed sideroblasts were not seen. Sucrose hemolysis and Ham's test were negative. Hepatitis B and C screening was negative. The antibody test for parvovirus was negative. Cytogenetic studies on the bone marrow showed an abnormal mosaic male pattern with del 5q, +8, and +11. All of these are recurring abnormalities in MDSs.

DIAGNOSIS: Hypoplastic RAEB.

CLINICAL COURSE: The patient was treated with cis-retinoic acid, folate, erythropoietin, and G-CSF, without any improvement. His blood counts have progressively worsened, and he is now dependent on packed red cell and platelet transfusions. In addition, he has developed frequent respiratory infections requiring intravenous antibiotics and hospitalization. He has refused chemotherapy. Because of his age, he is not a candidate for bone marrow transplantation.

DISCUSSION: There are two unique features to this case: hypoplasia of the bone marrow and the cytogenetic abnormalities. Bone marrow hypoplasia in this case is severe enough that a diagnosis of aplastic anemia could be entertained. However, unequivocal evidence for the presence of more than 5% blasts in the bone marrow clinches the diagnosis in favor of RAEB. The patient therefore has hypoplastic RAEB. The hypoplastic variants of MDSs form a distinct clinical entity and constitute about 16% of these cases. These are mostly seen in the RA, RARS, and RAEB subgroups. Occasionally, hypoplastic acute leukemia has also been reported. These patients have a poor prognosis because of their poor response to therapy and prolonged cytopenias after myeloablative treatment.

The hypoplastic MDSs have lower WBC and platelet counts and have macrocytic red cell indices. The prevalence of cytogenetic abnormalities, incidence of leukemic transformation, and survival are similar in the hypoplastic and normoplastic/hyperplastic MDSs. The response to therapy, whether directed at hypoplasia or myelodysplasia, is poor.

Over the last 15 years, there has been accumulating evidence of a large area of overlap between aplastic anemia and the MDSs (Chapter 9). Even in the early 1950s, it was recognized that 1 out of 35 patients with the diagnosis of aplastic anemia will evolve into myelodysplasia or acute leukemia. Similarly, PNH, a monoclonal stem cell disorder, can present with hypoplastic bone marrow and carries a distinct risk of transformation into acute leukemia. Over the last 10 years, many studies with large numbers of patients have reported that about a third of those with aplastic anemia will progress to MDSs, PNH, or acute leukemia over 10–15 years from the time of diagnosis. The reasons for this phenomenon are becoming somewhat clearer. It is possible that aplastic anemia in some patients starts as a clonal disorder. Evidence for this argument was provided by Van Kamp et al. (1991), who, in a study of 18 patients with acquired aplastic anemia, showed that 13 (72%) had clonal hematopoiesis. Clinical data appear to support this observation. Long-term follow-up of patients with aplastic anemia reveals that there is a 28% risk of developing a clonal hematopoietic disorder like PNH, MDS, or acute leukemia in the first 7 years after diagnosis. This risk increases to 42% in 10 years. Is the risk of developing monoclonal hematopoietic disorders in aplastic anemia worse now than it was in the 1950s? The answer to this question is not clear. It may be that the detection methods for disorders like PNH are better now than they were 40 years ago. Since most patients with aplastic anemia receive immunosuppressive therapy, it is possible that immunosuppression plays a role. However, there are no data to support these arguments.

Cytogenetic abnormalities affecting MDSs are discussed in detail in Chapter 7. From 50% to 60% of patients with primary MDSs have a cytogenetic abnormality. In secondary or t-MDSs, an abnormal karyotype may be seen in up to 86% of the patients. Chromosomal changes seen in primary MDSs are many (Table 7.1 in Chapter 7) and include the following common abnormalities: -7, $+8$, del 5, del 11q, del 12, del 13q, del 20q, t(1;3), t(2;11), t(6;9), and t(11;21). Chromosomal abnormalities seen in secondary or t-MDSs (Table 7.2 in Chapter 7) include the following: del(5q), del(7q), -5, -7, del(12p), t(1;7), $+8$, and $+21$. Even though changes involving chromosomes 5 and 7 are seen in primary as well as t-MDSs, these abnormalities are more typical of the latter. In some studies of patients with t-MDSs and acute leukemia, abnormalities involving chromosomes 5 and 7 constituted 94% of all karyotypic aberrations seen. Deletions involving 5q have been studied in great detail and involve band 5q31, termed the *critical region*. A number of genes have been mapped to this region and include genes for CD14, *EGR*1 gene, *PDGF* gene, adrenergic receptor protein gene, endothelial cell growth factor gene, and genes for IL-3, GM-CSF, IL-4, and IL-5. The relationship between 5q$-$ and the pathogenesis of MDSs seen with this lesion is not known. It is possible that this deletion leads to a loss of wild-type allele or a decrease in the gene product.

Chromosomal abnormalities provide useful prognostic information (see Chapters 2 and 9 for details of the scoring systems). In some studies, the cytogenetic abnormalities have been found to be of independent predictive value, while in others they do not supersede the blast percentage in the marrow. Some authors have combined the morphological features of the marrow and the cytogenetic abnormalities as a prognostic tool. At present, it is possible to divide the karyotypic abnormalities into three prognostically distinct groups. Patients with normal cytogenetic analysis or those with 5q− alone fall in the favorable group. These patients have a median survival of more than 2 years. Patients with trisomy 8 have an intermediate outlook, and median survival is 1–2 years. The third group, with the poorest outlook, includes patients with del 7 or multiple complex defects. The median survival in these patients is less than 1 year.

This patient thus has a primary hypoplastic MDS with a grim outlook. The presence of more than 5% blasts in the marrow and multiple cytogenetic abnormalities are the high-risk factors. Since allogeneic marrow transplantation is not possible and the patient has not responded to a differentiation-inducing agent or a CSF, his future therapy will have to be supportive.

SUMMARY

Morphology	Peripheral blood film: Immature, abnormal cells.
	Bone marrow aspirate: 17% blasts, agranular bands, and nuclear fragmentation. Iron stain +++, no ringed sideroblasts.
	Bone marrow biopsy: Hypoplasia with a fat:cell ratio of 90:10.
Cytochemistry	MPEX+, SBB+.
Cytogenetics	del 5q, +8, +11.
Sucrose hemolysis test	Negative.
Ham's test	Negative.
Hepatitis B and C serology	Negative.
Diagnosis	Hypoplastic RAEB.

ANSWERS

1. The diagnosis of RAEB with marrow hypoplasia can be made in this case on the basis of bone marrow morphology. The next most important study to be obtained is the cytogenetic analysis of the bone marrow. It provides information with diagnostic and prognostic significance.

2. Bone marrow hypoplasia is seen in about 16% of the patients with MDSs. It is very important that, in such cases, appropriate studies are performed to rule out PNH and aplastic anemia. As mentioned in the discussion, a significant number of patients with aplastic anemia have clonal hematopoiesis, and many patients develop clonal hematopoietic disorders 7–10 years after diagnosis. The hypoplastic group can also be treated with aplastic anemia regimens if the initial distinction between the diagnosis of aplastic anemia and MDS is blurred.

Patients with a clear-cut diagnosis of MDS, whether hypoplastic or not, have similar response rates to available therapies.

3. The most likely cause of frequent respiratory infections in this patient is neutrophil dysfunction. Many types of functional defects have been described in the neutrophils of patients with MDSs. These include myeloperoxidase deficiency, defects of degranulation, and decreased bactericidal activity.

BIBLIOGRAPHY

Articles

Boogaerts MA, Nelissen V, Roelant C, et al: Blood neutrophil function in primary myelodysplastic syndromes. *Br J Haematol* 55:217–227, 1983.

Breton-Gorius J, Houssay D, Vilde JL, et al: Partial myeloperoxidase deficiency in a case of preleukemia. II. Defects of degranulation and abnormal bactericidal activity of blood neutrophils. *Br J Haematol* 30:279–288, 1975.

de Bock R, de Jonge M, Korthout M, et al: Hypoplastic acute leukemia; description of eight cases and search for hematopoietic inhibiting activity. *Ann Hematol* 65:247–252, 1992.

DePlanque MM, Bacigalupo A, Wursch A, et al: Long term follow up of severe aplastic anemia patients treated with antithymocyte globulin. *Br J Haematol* 73:121–126, 1989.

De Witte T, Muus P, De Pauw B, et al: Intensive antileukemic treatment of patients younger than 65 years with myelodysplastic syndromes and secondary acute leukemia. *Cancer* 66:831–837, 1990.

Jacobs R, Cornbleet MA, Vardiman JW, et al: Prognostic implications of morphology and karyotype in primary myelodysplastic syndrome. *Blood* 67:1765–1772, 1986.

LeBeau MM, Albain KS, Larson RA, et al: Clinical and cytogenetic correlations in 63 patients with therapy related myelodysplastic syndromes and acute non-lymphocytic leukemia. Further evidence for characteristic abnormalities of chromosomes no. 5 and 7. *J Clin Oncol* 4:325–345, 1986.

LeBeau MM, Espinoza R, Neuman WL, et al: Cytogenetic and molecular delineation of the smallest commonly deleted region of chromosome 5 in malignant myeloid disease. *Proc Natl Acad Sci USA* 90:5484–5488, 1993.

Levine EG, Bloomfield CD: Secondary myelodysplastic syndromes and leukemias. *Clin Hematol* 15:1037–1080, 1986.

Mufti GJ: Chromosomal deletions in the myelodysplastic syndrome. *Leuk Res* 16:35–51, 1992.

Nand S, Godwin JG: Hypoplastic myelodysplastic syndrome. *Cancer* 62:958–964, 1964.

Ruutu P, Ruutu T, Vuopio P, et al: Function of neutrophils in preleukemia. *Scand J Haematol* 18:317–325, 1977.

van Kamp H, Landagent JE, Jansen JPM, et al: Clonal hematopoiesis in patients with acquired aplastic anemia. *Blood* 78:3209–3214, 1991.

Yunis JJ, Rydell RE, Oken MM, et al: Refined chromosome analysis as an independent prognostic indicator in de novo myelodysplastic syndromes. *Blood* 67:1721–1730, 1986.

Review Articles

Annotation: Is aplastic anemia a preleukemic disorder? *Br J Haematol* 77:447–452, 1991.

Berger R, Flandrin G: Chromosomal abnormalities in secondary acute myeloid leukemia and myelodysplastic syndromes. In Mufti GJ, Galton DAG (eds): *The Myelodysplastic Syndromes*. New York, Churchill Livingstone, 1992, pp 129–139.

Bloomfield CD: Chromosome abnormalities in secondary myelodysplastic syndromes. *Scand J Haematol* 36(Suppl 45):82–90, 1986.

Noel P, Tefferi A, Pierre RV, et al: Karyotypic analysis in primary myelodysplastic syndromes. *Blood Rev* 7:10–18, 1993.

CASE **8**

PATIENT: A 65-year-old Caucasian man.

CHIEF COMPLAINT: Abnormal hemogram.

MEDICAL HISTORY: The patient was admitted to the hospital after developing chest pain on the morning of admission. His CBC was found to be abnormal, and a hematology consultation was obtained. He had had hypertension for 8 years and underwent a colonoscopy 1 year ago, during which a small polyp was removed. He smoked one pack of cigarettes per day (37 pack-years) and drank about six beers a week. He was a machinist and denied exposure to unusual chemicals or radiation. His family history was unremarkable.

PHYSICAL EXAMINATION: The physical examination was normal.

LABORATORY RESULTS:

A. *Screening Procedure*
   WBC count was 11.9×10^9/L with 43% neutrophils, 17% lymphocytes, 39% monocytes, and 1% basophils. Hemoglobin was 12.4 g/dL, HCT 37.2%, MCV 93.2 fL, MCH 31.0 pg, MCHC 33.2 g/dL, and RDW 18.1%. The platelet count was 93×10^9/L. The chemistry profile was normal except for mild elevation of LDH at 224 IU/L (normal, 90–200 IU/L). Examination of the blood smear confirmed the presence of an increased number of monocytes (Case 8.1).

QUESTIONS

1. What is your diagnosis and why? What further investigations should now be undertaken?

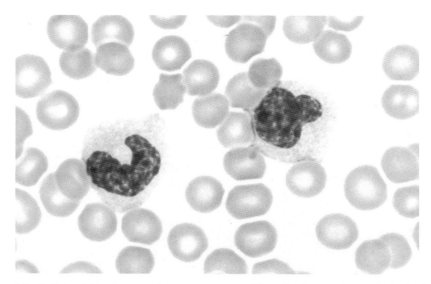

Case 8.1 Peripheral blood smear showing monocytes. Note the decreased granularity in the cytoplasm ($\times 1,000$).

2. Are the hematological abnormalities seen here responsible for the patient's chest pains?
3. What is the natural history of chronic myelomonocytic leukemia (CMML)? How does this disease differ from chronic granulocytic leukemia (CGL), and why are these two disorders classified in different categories (i.e., CMML is an MDS and CGL is an MPD) of disease?
4. How should this patient be treated?

LABORATORY RESULTS

B. *Confirmatory Studies*

Since monocytosis is also associated with chronic or granulomatous infections and malignancies, the patient was examined again, and a serial CBC was done to confirm the persistence of peripheral blood monocytosis. A bone marrow examination showed a fat:cell ratio of 40:60. A 200-cell differential count showed 8% blasts, 67% granulocytes, 14% erythroid cells, 2% monocytes, 1% plasma cells, 3% lymphocytes, and 5% promonocytes. Megakaryocytes were decreased and some appeared monolobular. Agranular bands, monocytes, and blast cells were seen on the aspirate smear (Case 8.2). Bone marrow biopsy showed large collections of monocytic cells (Case 8.3). Iron was decreased, and ringed sideroblasts were not seen. Cytochemical studies showed that the blasts were MPEX+, A-EST+ (fluoride sensitive), B-EST+, and C-EST+. Bone marrow was sent for cytogenetic analysis, which showed a normal male karyotype.

DIAGNOSIS: CMML.

CLINICAL COURSE: Oral folate and cis-retinoic acid therapy was begun for the CMML, and the patient's angina was managed conservatively. Five months after his diagnosis, the patient started to experience easy fatigue. The physical

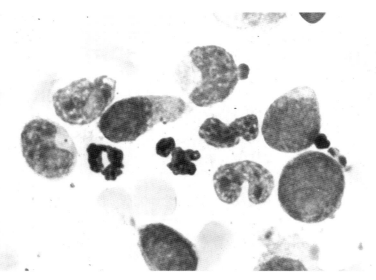

Case 8.2   Bone marrow aspirate showing blast cells, agranular bands, and monocytes (×1,000).

examination was normal. CBC showed a WBC count of $6.0 \times 10^9/L$, with 53% neutrophils, 34% lymphocytes, and 13% monocytes. Hemoglobin was 10.2 g/dL, and the platelet count was $55 \times 10^9/L$. Bone marrow examination showed 13% blasts, 3% promonocytes, 49% granulocytic precursors, 25% erythroid precursors, and 10% lymphocytes. In another 6 weeks, the fatigue had become disabling and a bone marrow test was repeated. The blast count had now increased to 30%. The blasts were MPEX+, SBB+, B-EST+, A-EST+ and sensitive to fluoride and weakly positive for PAS, supporting the diagnosis of M5a AML. The patient was hospital-

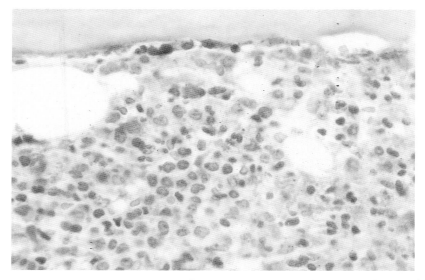

Case 8.3   Bone marrow biopsy specimen showing an aggregation of monocytic elements (×400).

ized and given induction chemotherapy with high-dose cytarabine. On day 23, he died of septic complications.

DISCUSSION: This patient had CMML which evolved into AML in about 7 months. The diagnostic criteria for CMML (Table 2.1, Chapter 2) are as follows: peripheral blood showing monocytosis of more than 10^9/L, peripheral blood blasts less than 5%, and absence of Auer rods. The bone marrow shows variable trilineage dysplasia, and the blast count is less than 5% but occasionally may be 5–20%. Frequently, an increase in monocytic precursors is observed.

The first description of CMML was published in 1972 by Zittoun et al., and the FAB group included it as a subgroup of MDSs in 1982. The median age at diagnosis is 66 years, and males are affected more often (male:female ratio is 2.4:1). Splenomegaly is present in about half of the patients and may become massive in some. Chromosomal abnormalities are found in about 34% of those studied and commonly are trisomy 8, del 7, del 20, t(1;3), and t(5;12). The median survival for patients with CMML is quite variable, ranging from 2 months to 3 years. The risk of leukemic transformation also varies between 16% and 34% in different studies. Analysis of risk factors in CMML yields results similar to those seen in other FAB subgroups. In a study from the Mayo Clinic (Teffer, 1989), only the marrow blast percentage was an independent prognostic variable. A French study (Feneax 1988) of 107 patients with CMML showed that a marrow blast percentage of more than 5%, low hemoglobin level, and leukocytosis were adverse prognostic factors.

Recently, the molecular genetics of CMML patients with t(5;12) have been studied further, with interesting results. This translocation leads to fusion between a member of the *ETS* family of transcription factors named *TEL* and platelet-derived growth factor receptor (PDGFR) beta. The altered PDGFR beta can cause deregulation of *RAS* mechanisms, thereby adding to the accumulating body of evidence that *RAS* abnormalities may be central to the pathogenesis of many myeloid leukemias.

At times, the distinction between CMML and CGL becomes difficult on clinical grounds, especially if the patients have high WBC counts. The marrow cytogenetics are very helpful in pinpointing the diagnosis, as the vast majority (95%) of CGL patients show the presence of the Philadelphia (Ph') chromosome. The real difficulty arises in patients with so-called Ph'-negative CGL. Some of these patients have been shown to have the *bcr-abl* rearrangement by more sensitive techniques. When the *BCR-ABL* translocation cannot be demonstrated, there is real doubt about the diagnosis of CGL, and many investigators believe that such patients have an MDS rather than CGL. If the diagnostic criteria for CMML are met in such patients, it is the likeliest diagnosis. Some investigators feel that Ph'-negative CGL and CMML are variants of the same disease.

Activating *RAS* mutations are very common in CMML and have been described in 20–80% of these patients. In contrast, the incidence of *RAS* mutations is very low in CGL, occurring in 1–3% of patients. *RAS* mutations are also associated with a higher rate of progression to acute leukemia and poor survival. Thus, *RAS* mutations may help in differentiating CMML from Ph'-negative CGL and may provide the clinician with important prognostic information.

Occasionally, CMML may be confused with myeloproliferative disorders other than CGL. This may happen in patients with early-phase myelofibrosis with myeloid metaplasia (MMM) and patients with polycythemia vera with high WBC counts. The distinction, however, is easily made. In the latter two disorders, absence of monocytosis, lack of dysplastic changes in the marrow, high hemoglobin level, and normal to high platelet counts help distinguish them from CMML. The late stages of MMM may be associated with cytopenias due to massive splenomegaly, but they are not known to be associated with monocytosis.

Predictably, the response to available therapies in CMML has been similar to that seen in other subgroups of MDSs, and the same therapeutic guidelines (Chapter 9) should be followed in treating these patients. Whenever possible, allogeneic bone marrow transplantation should be considered. Occasionally, unique clinical situations may arise requiring specific interventions. A patient with painful splenomegaly may require splenic irradiation or chemotherapy. Hydroxyurea and busulfan have been tried in patients with high WBC counts, with good short-term palliation.

SUMMARY

Morphology	**Peripheral blood film: Increased number of monocytes in the peripheral blood smear.** **Bone marrow aspirate: 8% blasts, agranular bands at the time of diagnosis.** **Later aspirates showed 30% blasts.**
Bone marrow cytochemistry	**MPEX+, A-EST+, A-EST (fluoride sensitive), B-EST+, C-EST (CAE−, A-EST+).**
Cytogenetics	**46,XY.**
Chemistry profile	**Elevated LDH.**
Diagnosis	**CMML (with subsequent transformation to AML-M5a).**

ANSWERS

1. The diagnosis at presentation was CMML, not RAEB. Even though the patient had more than 5% blasts in the marrow, monocytosis remained a prominent and persistent feature of his disease. The marrow in CMML, according to the diagnostic criteria set up by the FAB group, usually has less than 5% blasts but may occasionally have up to 20% blasts (Chapter 2). Those with 20–30% blasts have been referred to as having CMML in transformation (CMML-IT).

2. It is unlikely that the hematological abnormalities are responsible for the angina in this patient. His hemoglobin level is high enough for adequate oxygen delivery, and the normal WBC count is unlikely to cause complications from leukostasis. Therefore, in all likelihood, the angina is unrelated to the hematologic problems.

3. CMML is an aggressive subgroup of the MDSs and is generally associated with a poor prognosis. The disease primarily affects patients in the seventh decade, and males are affected about 2.5 times as often as females. Splenomegaly is seen in about half of these patients. Leukemic transformation occurs in about one-third of the patients. Median survival varies greatly in published reports, with a range of 2 months to 3 years. When data from large series are combined, the average survival of these patients seems to be about 11 months.

CMML can look remarkably similar to CGL at times. Splenomegaly and a left shift of the granulocytic series, though more common in CGL, can be seen in CMML. Monocytosis remains a unique feature of CMML, but it should be remembered that monocytosis can occur with prolonged bacterial infections, granulomatous infections, and various cancers. If there is a clinical suspicion of any such condition, it should be ruled out first. CMML is distinguished from CGL mainly by cytogenetics. If the patient is shown to have the Ph' chromosome, or a *BCR-ABL* rearrangement by the PCR or FISH technique, the diagnosis of CGL is secure. If the patient is shown to have cytogenetic abnormalities associated with CMML, it is likely CMML. Patients with normal cytogenetics may pose a diagnostic dilemma. Could these be the so-called Ph'-negative CGL? However, many investigators believe that there may be no such entity and that all these patients may actually have an MDS. As mentioned in the discussion, *RAS* mutations, seen rarely in CGL, have been described in 20–80% of patients with CMML. *RAS* mutations impart a poor prognosis to this group, with higher rates of leukemic transformation and short survival.

The reasons for classifying CGL as an MPD and CMML as an MDS are subtle. The bone marrow in CGL is almost always hyperplastic. In CMML, it may be normoplastic or hyperplastic. Evidence for hematopoietic dysplasia is much more likely to be seen in CMML than in CGL, where morphologically the marrow cells look normal. But both disorders are distinctly pre-acute leukemic; leukemic transformation occur in about 75% of patients with CGL compared to only 34% in CMML.

4. Since the diagnosis of CMML was made accidentally, and since the CBC values were within the safe range, initial therapy with nontoxic agents in this patient was justified. However, these agents did not prove to be of help. After he transformed into acute leukemia, the only choice was to give him chemotherapy; bone marrow transplantation could not be done because of his age and his cardiac problems. Unfortunately, the patient died of sepsis, the most common complication seen in such patients.

BIBLIOGRAPHY

Articles

Alessandrino EP, Orlandi E, Brusamolino E, et al: Chronic myelomonocytic leukemia. Clinical features, cytogenetics and prognosis in 30 consecutive cases. *Hematol Oncol* 3:147–155, 1985.

Bartram CR: Molecular genetic aspects of myelodysplastic syndromes. In Koeffler HP (ed): *Myelodysplastic Syndromes*. Philadelphia, WB Saunders, 1992, pp 557–570.

Bennet JM, Catovsky D, Daniel MT, et al: The French American British (FAB) Co-operative Group. Proposals for classification of myelodysplastic syndromes. *Br J Haematol* 51:189–199, 1982.

Fenaux P, Beuscart R, Lai JL, et al: Prognostic factors in adult chronic myelomonocytic leukemia. An analysis of 107 cases. *J Clin Oncol* 6:1417–1424, 1988.

Golub TR, Barker GF, Lovett M, et al: Fusion of PDGF receptor beta to a novel *ets*-like gene, *tel*, in chronic myelomonocytic leukemia with t(5;12) chromosomal translocation. *Cell* 77:307–312, 1994.

Hirsch-Ginsberg C, LeMaistre AC, Kantarjian H, et al: *RAS* mutations are rare events in Ph' negative/*bcr* negative chronic myelogenous leukemia, but are prevalent in chronic myelomonocytic leukemia. *Blood* 76:1214–1219, 1990.

Martiat P, Michaux JL, Rodhain J. Ph' negative chronic myeloid leukemia. Comparison with Ph' positive chronic myeloid leukemia and chronic myelomonocytic leukemia. The Groupe Français de Cytogentique Hematologique. *Blood* 78:205–211, 1991.

Ribera JM, Cervantes F, Rozman C: A multivariate analysis of prognostic factors in chronic myelomonocytic leukemia according to the FAB criteria. *Br J Haematol* 65:307–311, 1987.

Tefferi A, Hoagland HC, Therneau TM, et al: Chronic myelomonocytic leukemia. Natural history and prognostic determinants. *Mayo Clin Proc* 64:1246–1254, 1989.

Todd WM, Pierre RV: Preleukemia: A long term prospective study of 326 patients. *Scand J Haematol* 36:114–120, 1986.

Travis LB, Pierre RV, DeWald GW: Ph'-negative chronic granulocytic leukemia: A nonentity. *Am J Clin Pathol* 85:186–193, 1986.

Urbano-Ispizua A, Gill R, Matutes E, et al: Low frequency of *ras* oncogene mutations in Ph' positive acute leukemia and a report of a novel mutation H61 Leu in a single case. *Leukemia* 6:342–346, 1992.

Zittoun R, Bernadou A, Bilski PG, et al: Les leucemies myelomonocytaires subaigues. Etude de 27 cas et revue de la litterature. *Semin Hop Paris* 48:1943–1956, 1972.

Review Articles

Beris P: Primary clonal myelodysplastic syndromes. *Semin Hematol* 26:216–233, 1989.

Cheson BD: Chemotherapy and bone marrow transplantation for myelodysplastic syndromes. *Semin Oncol* 19:106–114, 1992.

Galton DAG: Haematological differences between chronic granulocytic leukemia, atypical chronic granulocytic leukemia, and chronic myelomonocytic leukemia. *Leuk- Lymphoma* 7:343–350, 1992.

Ganser A, Hoelzer D: Clinical course of myelodysplastic syndromes. *Hematol Oncol Clin North Am* 6:607–632, 1992.

Heim S: Cytogenetic findings in primary and secondary myelodysplastic syndromes. *Leuk Res* 16:43–46, 1992.

Mecucci C, Van den Berghe H: Cytogenetics. *Hematol Oncol Clin North Am* 6:523–542, 1992.

INDEX